The Prevention of Cancer

The Prevention of Cancer
Pointers from Epidemiology

Richard Doll

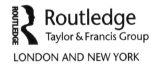

Routledge
Taylor & Francis Group

LONDON AND NEW YORK

First published 1967 by Transaction Publishers

Published 2017 by Routledge
2 Park Square, Milton Park, Abingdon, Oxon OX14 4RN
711 Third Avenue, New York, NY 10017, USA

Routledge is an imprint of the Taylor & Francis Group, an informa business

Library of Congress Catalog Number: 2008002632

Library of Congress Cataloging-in-Publication Data
Doll, Richard.
  The prevention of cancer : pointers from epidemiology / Richard Doll.
      p. ; cm.
  Originally published: London : Nuffield Provincial Hospitals Trust, 1967.
  Includes bibliographical references and index.
  ISBN 978-0-202-36220-5 (alk. paper)
  1. Cancer—Prevention. 2. Cancer—Epidemiology. I. Title.
  [DNLM: 1. Neoplasms—epidemiology. 2. Neoplasm—prevention & control. QZ 200 D665p 1967a]

RC268.D6 2008
614.5'999--dc22   2008002632

ISBN 13: 978-0-202-36220-5 (pbk)

The Rock Carling Fellowship was founded as an annual memorial to the late Sir Ernest Rock Carling, for many years a Governing Trustee if the Nuttfield Provincial Hospitals Trust and Chairman of the Trust's Medical Advisory Committee. Each holder of the fellowship will seek to review in a monograph the state of knowledge and activity in one of the fields in which Sir Ernest had been particularly interested and which is within the purposes of the Trust. The arrangements provide that the monograph will be introduced by a public lecture to be given at a recognized medical teaching centre in the United Kingdom.

CONTENTS

Chapter 1

INTRODUCTION

When, some fifteen years ago, a professor of surgery told me that it was not only a waste of time but also faintly immoral to try to prevent cancer, he had in mind the idea that the development of cancer was part of the normal process of ageing. Attempts to interfere with it were, at best, doomed to failure. At worst they represented the sort of *lèse-majesté* which Prometheus was guilty of, and were liable to lead to some comparable retribution. This view was not, I hope, widely held; but it represented, in extreme form, a fatalistic attitude that was. So little was known about the nature of malignant cells and of the processes that normally regulate tissue growth, that the prevention of cancer, regarded as theoretically possible, was not thought to be a practicable current objective. Medical education and public hopes were, therefore, concentrated on methods of improving treatment and of diagnosing the disease at an early stage, when treatment might be more effective.

Since then the situation has altered radically. New classes of chemical carcinogens have been discovered, some of which occur naturally in the human environment and are capable of causing experimental cancer in organs that were previously difficult to affect. It is now known, for example, that nitrosamines, given by mouth, will readily produce cancer of the oesophagus, stomach or large bowel. Fungi, like Aspergillus flavus, have been shown to produce metabolites in foodstuffs stored under hot and humid conditions, minute doses of which will produce cancer of the liver and the stomach. The pyrrolizidine alkaloids in Senecio and other plant families have been found to produce cancer of the liver, and the cycad nut to contain a substance that is potentially capable of producing carcinoma of the large bowel. The nut is only an occasional food for man, but the discovery of cycasin, its active principle, may be of far-reaching importance; for it provides an example of a substance that is harmless in itself but which gives rise to a carcinogen in the bowel of an animal with a normal intestinal flora. And overshadowing all this is the discovery that viruses can produce cancer in so many species of animals that it is difficult not to believe that they can also produce some types of cancer in man.

Pari passu with these developments, epidemiological studies have shown that cancer incidence in man is far more dependent on the conditions of his life than had previously been supposed. The few classical examples of cancers that occurred with heavy exposure to a specific occupational hazard, or were associated with such bizarre habits as smoking a cigar with the burning end inside the mouth, have been steadily added to; and in some instances it has been possible to show that the incidence of cancer falls when the method of work or the associated habit is changed. Variation in incidence is, moreover, now known to be the rule rather than the exception. No cancer that occurs with even moderate frequency, occurs everywhere and always to the same extent. A range of ten or twentyfold is common and for some types of cancer it is far wider. Sometimes it has even been possible to recognize an epidemic, similar in scale to an epidemic of infectious disease, but modified by the fact that the induction period may be of the order of thirty years.

A change in attitude has, therefore, occurred and the prevention of cancer is now coming to be regarded as a practicable alternative to its cure. We are, however, still almost totally ignorant of the mechanism by which cancer is produced at the cellular level and, until we know this, our methods of prevention are liable to be cumbersome and inefficient. Ethical considerations and the time scale of the disease make it impossible to obtain experimental evidence in man, and we have to decide what action to take from observation of Nature's experiments and by analogy from experiments in animals.

Of these two sources of evidence, that derived from animal experiments offers the most obvious advantages. The range of possibilities is enormous and the imagination of the investigator can be given free rein; moreover, by good design and sufficiently frequent repetition it is possible to be virtually certain of the relationship between cause and effect. Animal experimentation has, however, the disadvantage that an exact recreation of the relevant human conditions may not be possible and the necessary limitation on numbers makes it difficult to study the effect of small doses and of weakly carcinogenic agents. Analogy, moreover, is an uncertain guide. Animals vary greatly in their susceptibility to cancer induction, and an agent that is highly carcinogenic in one species may have little or no effect in another. Methylcholanthrene, for example, is a most powerful carcinogen, yet it's activity would probably have been passed over if it had been tested originally in apes; and arsenic, which is certainly carcinogenic to man, has never been shown to produce cancer in any other species.

In these circumstances, the evidence from epidemiological studies is of particular interest. Relationships may be suggested that would never be thought of in the ordinary course of laboratory work and the results of such studies are directly relevant to the problems of human disease. Moreover, the large numbers at risk and the intensity of the medical care to which man is subjected, make it possible to recognize relatively small effects. There is, however, the disadvantage that it may be extremely difficult to decide what a particular relationship means, and to differentiate a real effect from a secondary and unimportant epiphenomenon. Despite this difficulty, the observation of Nature's experiments has contributed a great deal to knowledge about cancer. Practical decisions, based on information thus obtained, have largely eliminated the risk of cancer due to occupational hazards in several industries, and there is no reason to suppose that similar action in other fields will not be equally effective.

Chapter 2

THE NATURE OF EPIDEMIOLOGICAL
EVIDENCE

Epidemiological studies contribute to the prevention of cancer in three main ways. First, by demonstrating differences in the incidence of cancer in different communities and correlating them with differences in the prevalence of a potential aetiological factor, it may become possible to suggest a new clue to its cause. Secondly, hypotheses about the cause of cancer can be tested by relating the occurrence of the disease to a personal characteristic of the affected individuals – either to their constitution or to the degree to which they have been exposed to an environmental agent. Thirdly, the reality of a causal relationship can be put to the acid test of practice, by seeing whether the disease can be prevented by changing the prevalence of the suspected agent.

Of these three methods, the first has been used most intensively, and it might be thought that all the important differences had already been discovered. In the field of cancer, however, this is most unlikely. Large parts of the world have only recently been opened up to medical research and there is still very little quantitative information about the incidence of any type of cancer outside Europe and North America. Moreover, even when we know that a cancer varies in incidence, we may have no knowledge of the boundary between the high and low incidence areas (as, for example, with cancer of the liver in Mozambique and cancer of the stomach in the Kivu region of the Congo), and it is just this knowledge that is likely to be most helpful in correlating incidence with the appropriate carcinogenic factor. We are also gradually realizing that cancer varies almost as much in time as in space, and that the recent pandemic of lung cancer is only an extreme example of a process that is characteristic of nearly all cancers, some forms of the disease becoming more common while others are disappearing. During the past few years, developments in experimental oncology have indicated many more classes of carcinogens, so that there is now more opportunity than ever before for discovering new correlations.

The characteristic feature of this type of study is, however, that information is obtained about communities as a whole and not about individuals. Evidence of an association (for example, between the average duration of lactation and the incidence of cancer of the breast) is, therefore, indirect and though it may be extremely valuable in suggesting a hypothesis for detailed study by other methods, definite conclusions about aetiology cannot be drawn from it. It must also be remembered that few, if any, cancers have only one cause, that the causes may interact with one another, and that the estimates of individual exposure that can be obtained from national data are, at best, extremely crude. A correlation co-efficient of the order of 0·5 between mortality rates and the prevalence of a particular agent in different countries must, in these circumstances, be regarded as good evidence that the agent *may* be involved in the production of the disease, but whether it is or is not must be determined by other evidence of an entirely different type.

To this further evidence, epidemiology can make an

important contribution by the carefully designed collection of observations on individual subjects and a detailed statistical analysis of the results. Two methods have been commonly used – the retrospective, starting from affected patients and unaffected controls, and the prospective, starting from subjects with varying degrees of exposure to the agent under study. Both methods have their advantages and disadvantages; but neither can overcome completely the difficulty that any relationship that is found may be a secondary one and that the suspected agent may itself be associated with another which is, in fact, the true carcinogen.

In recent years much epidemiological evidence of this type has been collected and a great deal of time and energy have been spent in arguing about its meaning. Does it, for example, prove that exposure to diagnostic radiography in utero causes childhood cancer, that circumcision of the husband will prevent cancer of the cervix uteri, or that the possession of the blood group A antigen predisposes to the development of cancer of the salivary glands, stomach and pancreas? Some commentators have tried to set up criteria comparable to Koch's postulates in the field of bacteriology, which would act as guide lines to a correct conclusion. The objective is worthy; but I wonder whether it is really practicable? As Bradford Hill said: 'I am not convinced that we can. . . reduce a wide variety of complex situations to a simple common denominator – that is, to one that can be really useful and not merely state the obvious. I am not convinced that we can in advance decide what weight we shall give to this or that piece of evidence.'

Consider, for example, the Kangri cancer of the skin of the lower abdomen and thighs, found among the Kashmiri who warm themselves in winter by carrying, in front of their abdomen and suspended from the neck, an earthen pot full of live coals, or the 'chutta cancer' of the hard palate, found in Vizagapatam among those who are accustomed to holding a homemade cigar with the lighted end inside the mouth to prevent it going out. These associations have not been demonstrated by detailed retrospective studies of patients and controls, nor by prospective studies of persons with and without the specific habits, such as have been reported for some other cancers. Nevertheless a few case histories and the close geographical association between the local habits and the occurrence of the disease have sufficed to convince nearly all who have been interested in the subject that the relationships are causal. How much, I wonder, has the readiness with which these conclusions have been accepted been influenced by the fact that few European or American oncologists are in the habit of carrying a heated pot close to their abdomen in winter, or of smoking their cigars outside in?

According to Berkson, we can conclude that an observed association indicates cause and effect only under strictly limited conditions. In his words: 'If an essential biological association is to be established as a definite scientific conclusion, that is to say, if it is to be considered "proved" the population must not be anything else, except an experimental population. An association found in a purely statistical investigation made on an existent population, by which I mean an investigation which is retrospective as regards either of the variables concerned, however strongly it may suggest association as a presumptive conclusion, is tentative until it is corroborated fully by means of experiment.' And he goes on to explain that by association he means here a necessary biological relationship or, if I understand him correctly, a relationship between cause and effect.

There can, I think, be no serious disagreement with this formulation of Berkson's. Some people might maintain on philosophical grounds that even under these conditions it was improper to speak of 'proof' – I know an eminent mathematical statistician who holds that one cannot be certain that the sun will rise tomorrow – but this is, I think, irrelevant to the practical scientific problem. If then we accept Berkson's dictum, what effect does it have on our interpretation of epidemiological data?

Consider the problem of the carcinogenic effect of small doses of X-rays on the foetus in utero. The first suggestion that there might be a measurable effect came in 1956 when Stewart, Webb and Hewitt reported that more of the mothers of children who had died of cancer before the age of ten years said that they had been subjected to radiographic examination of the abdomen during the relevant pregnancy than of a selected group of mothers whose children had survived. The reality of the difference was subsequently confirmed by MacMahon using a somewhat different technique. In MacMahon's study the birth certificates of all the children who had died of cancer in certain States were traced and those children who had been born in hospital were selected for special study. The frequency with which the mothers of these children had been X-rayed during their pregnancies was determined by examination of the hospital notes, and the results were compared with those obtained for a one per cent random sample of children born in the same hospitals during the same period. By Berkson's criterion it is evident that neither study can prove that diagnostic X-rays were the cause of the cancer; in both cases the women were irradiated (or said they had been irradiated) for reasons over which the observer had no control, and it is impossible to rule out the possibility that the cancer was connected with the reason for which they were X-rayed and not with the radiography itself.

How then can we prove the relationship is causal? The evidence would certainly be strengthened if it were shown that a similar effect had been produced experimentally in several different animal species; but the practical difficulties of maintaining, treating, following and examining an animal population of the size, perhaps 50,000, required to demonstrate so small an effect are so enormous that it is not surprising that no such evidence is available. Even if it were, an element of doubt would still remain as to whether the results were applicable to man. We are left, therefore, with the conclusion that proof can be obtained only by means of human experiment, which, though not impossible to conceive in this situation, is certainly not ethical to carry out. In practice it is unlikely that we shall get much more certain evidence than we now have – at least until we have obtained a complete understanding of the way in which radiation induces cancer. Meanwhile decisions will have to be taken, both from the point of view of the public health and of further research, on the basis of evidence that is admittedly short of proof.

The practical question is, therefore, how to decide if the observed data are most reasonably explained on the basis of a cause and effect relationship. In the final analysis, the decision will inevitably be a matter for subjective judgement, but there are certain steps on the way to the decision that all would wish to take. The first is the demonstration that the association between factor and disease is real and not an artefact produced by the method of inquiry; that is, one or other of Yerushalmy and Palmer's first two criteria must be met, namely:

1. that the suspected characteristic is found more frequently in persons with the disease in question than in persons without the disease; or

2. that persons possessing the characteristic develop the disease more frequently than persons not possessing the characteristic.

To decide that the results of a particular study meet these criteria, we shall have recourse to the following considerations.

The most obvious is that the results should be repeatable. The same broad answer obtained in different places at different times by different workers is more impressive than a single unsupported observation. It is true, as Berkson has stressed, that repetition of the same error will produce the same fallacious results, so that repetition is not in itself a guarantee of validity. Nevertheless, if failure to repeat the results weighs against the reality of the association, it follows that repetition must add some weight in its favour.

The value of repetition may be further enhanced if in addition the hypothesis can be investigated by means of a different technique. For example, the fact that retrospective studies of patients with and without lung cancer and prospective studies of persons of different smoking habit indicated such similar quantitative relationships (Doll and Hill, 1954) weighed heavily in favour of their reality. Both types of study were open to bias, but the types of bias were different, and it would have been a remarkable coincidence if both had produced similar but yet spurious results.

And here we have arrived at the heart of the problem. The results may have been reproducible, and similar results may have been obtained by different techniques, and yet they may all have been produced by various types of bias. There is, unfortunately, no easy method by which this possibility can be automatically excluded. The only safeguard is always to suspect the influence of bias, consider every way it could have entered the study and then test to see if it has. In this respect, each investigation is a rule to itself, new possibilities being introduced with every variation in methodology and with the individual characteristics of the cases concerned.

In MacMahon's study, for example, there was one possibility of bias in that the data for some of the affected children were collected after the control data were complete; and it was this group of children, who had died most recently and who were in the older age group, who contributed the greater part of the excess history of radiation. It was, therefore, possible that the worker who extracted the records had become more efficient as time went on and had succeeded in tracing more references to irradiation in the later part of the series than in the earlier. This possibility was excluded by giving the investigator a randomly selected sample of the control and cancer series to re-examine at the end of the study, without his knowing which case was the control. In the event, he missed one X-ray record and traced another in both groups, so that the type of bias suspected was unlikely to have been an adequate explanation of the facts.

In the retrospective study of lung cancer that Sir Austin Bradford Hill and I carried out many types of bias were considered, but at least one possibility was overlooked*. It is possible that patients presenting with cough were admitted to hospital at an earlier stage of their disease than those without, so that those with cough (who might be expected to have been heavier smokers than average) might have survived longer after admission and might, therefore, have been more readily available for interview. In fact, this proved not to have influenced the results, but it was an interesting idea and certainly worth investigating.

Sometimes it is possible to exclude bias by reference to histology. For many types of cancer there is reason to believe that the different histological types have different causes. Adenocarcinoma and other types of bronchial carcinoma, chronic myeloid and chronic lymphatic leukaemia, transitional and squamous cell carcinoma of the bladder, and basal and squamous cell carcinoma of the skin provide examples. Most of these conditions can be studied as a single entity, the histological classification being made after the data have been collected. Few forms of bias are likely to distinguish between the different histological types, so that is usually safe to conclude that a relationship which holds only for some histological types of the disease and not for others is likely to be real.

To show that the association is real is, of course, the

* Doll and Hill, 1952.

first and easier step. It remains to decide whether the association is causal, or whether the factor and the disease are related to one another only because they are both related to something else. In distinguishing between these alternatives, we are likely to be influenced by many considerations:

1. The first, and in some ways the most important, is the strength of the relationship; that is, the ratio between the incidence of the disease among persons with and without the factor. The value of this ratio has been described in detail by Cornfield and Haenszel. Its use has, however, been the subject of criticism by Berkson who suggested that the absolute increase is more important. This criticism is, I think, due to a misunderstanding of the purpose for which the ratio is used. It is true that a small proportional increase in the incidence of a common disease may be more important, from the point of view of the public health, than a large proportional increase in the incidence of a rare disease. It would be a matter of much greater concern if an agent doubled the incidence of cancer of the large bowel than if it quadrupled the risk of cancer of the small intestine. That is, if one were certain that the agent was, in fact, responsible for the increase in both. But, from the point of view of determining aetiology the size of the proportional increase is of much greater significance than the size of the increase in absolute numbers. The best evidence of all is that which describes the conditions under which all cases of the disease occur. The fact that African childhood lymphoma was thought to be confined to persons who live in parts of Africa where the temperature never falls below 16°C was compelling epidemiological evidence of the

existence of a local agent; it is quite irrelevant to this evidence that the total number of cases is small*. Such an extreme situation is unusual. But it is not uncommon to find an incidence of ten or twenty-fold among exposed persons compared with an unexposed control group and it is much less easy to explain an increase of this order of magnitude as an incidental finding than it is to explain an increase of less than double.

2. The second characteristic is the existence of a biological gradient; that is, a quantitative gradation between the incidence of the disease and the dose of the factor. Cancer of the cervix uteri, for example, is known to occur more frequently among married women than among single, and among women who have borne children than among those who have not. Both factors are clearly inter-related so that each must be taken into account when assessing the effect of the other. When this is done the estimated risk is found to increase steadily with decreasing age at first marriage, whereas there is no similar increase with increase in the number of pregnancies: and this is good evidence that the agent is linked with marriage *per se* rather than with childbearing.

3. The third consideration – the specificity of the relationship – has been emphasized by Berkson and by Yerushalmy and Palmer. In the words of the latter, 'An observed association. . .must be tested for validity by investigating the relationship between the characteristic and other diseases and, if possible, the relationship of similar or

* In fact the disease is now known to occur in Europe and North America, but it is so rare in these areas that the argument is scarcely altered.

related characteristics to the disease in question. The suspected characteristic can be said to be specifically related to the disease. . .when. . .similar relationships do not exist with a variety of characteristics and with many disease entities when such relationships are not predictable on physiologic, pathologic, experimental or epidemiologic grounds. . .'

A good example of the use of this criterion is given by Yerushalmy. Several investigators have reported that the birth-weight of the child is negatively correlated with the mother's smoking habits and have suggested that a relatively low birth-weight is directly due to the mother's smoking. Yerushalmy found a similar correlation with the father's smoking habits arguing, correctly if his data were typical, that this lack of specificity suggested both relationships were more likely to be coincidental than causal.

The criterion, as put forward by Yerushalmy and Palmer, is complex and it will be noted that it contains a number of qualifications; I will refer later to the question of what can be regarded as biologically predictable, but, apart from this, at least two other qualifications need to be added. The first is that the environmental conditions responsible for human disease may act as vectors for more than one specific agent and they may affect different organs in different ways: Cornfield and his colleagues cited the effect of the London smog of 1952, as one example, and Bradford Hill cited polluted milk which could be responsible for such disparate diseases as tuberculosis, typhoid, diphtheria, scarlet fever, dysentery and undulant fever. It is clearly unreasonable to suppose that a complex agent need be related to only one disease.

The second is the need to take account of the degree of the association as well as the fact of its existence. Lilienfeld has pointed out that an agent may be related to different diseases for different reasons and the existence of some incidental relationships does not exclude the possibility that others are causal. In particular one cannot conclude that a close association is incidental solely because this is the most likely explanation for several minor relationships.

4. A fourth consideration is the extent to which the data fit with other epidemiological evidence. Tests may be made to see whether differences in incidence between the sexes, between countries, and within one country at different periods, correspond with differences in the prevalence of the agent; but the results of such tests must be interpreted with caution. For example, several commentators have argued that the increase in the ratio of the male and female mortality rates from lung cancer which continued in many countries throughout the 1950's was incompatible with the hypothesis that cigarette smoking caused the disease, because the consumption of cigarettes had increased much more among women than among men. Examination of the data in greater detail showed, however, that the trend in the sex ratio varied greatly with age and that when this was taken into account the apparent discrepancy disappeared (Springett, 1966).

5. Fifthly, we must ask whether the suspected causation is biologically plausible; whether one can visualize a mechanism through which it could work, and whether it accords with animal experiments and with any independent clinical and pathological observations. Important though this is, we should not, however, press it too far. To quote

Bradford Hill again: 'There was no biological knowledge to support (or to refute) Pott's observation in the eighteenth century of the excess of cancer in chimney sweeps. It was lack of biological knowledge in the nineteenth century that led a prize essayist writing on the value and the fallacy of statistics to conclude, amongst other "absurd" associations, that "it could be no more ridiculous for the stranger who passed the night in the steerage of an emigrant ship to ascribe the typhus, which he there contracted, to the vermin with which the bodies of the sick might be infected." And, coming to nearer times in the twentieth century there was no biological knowledge to support the evidence against rubella,' as a teratogenic agent. No field of knowledge is as yet complete and the observation of a new relationship may prove to be the beginning of a new series of observations rather than the culmination of an old.

6. Finally, after taking all these considerations into account, we shall have to return to the fundamental question – and ask whether any alternative hypothesis can explain the observations equally well or better. Sometimes the alternative hypothesis can be put to the test. When it was suggested that the association between intrauterine irradiation and childhood cancer arose because some feature in the mother-child complex predisposed to both, MacMahon could answer that he had examined toxaemia of pregnancy, disproportion, forceps delivery and several other features, and that none of them could explain the results, but he could not claim to have examined every feature of pregnancy and it might be that he had failed to recognize the only one that was really relevant. In the final analysis the answer to this, as to all other similar

questions, is largely a matter of personal judgement and scientific taste.

Epidemiology, however, need not always leave us in this unsatisfactory position; often we can try the experiment by removing the suspected agent and observing the result. Even when this is not practicable (the suspected agent being constitutional, or as ineradicable as sexual inter-course), or, if practicable, impossible to carry through as a controlled experiment, nevertheless something can still be gained. Few would doubt, for example, that the dis-appearance of carcinoma of the scrotum from among cotton spinners after the substitution of other lubricating oils for shale oil, or of carcinoma of the back of the hands among radiologists after they took to wearing leaded gloves, was conclusive evidence that shale oil and X-rays were carcinogenic to the skin of man. The difficulty is that the experiment may be expensive in energy and money, and it may need the co-operation of many people who have to be convinced that the experiment will be successful before it can even be begun.

Chapter 3

THE GEOGRAPHICAL AND TEMPORAL
DISTRIBUTION

Statistical aspects

The potential value of studies of the distribution of cancer
as providing a source of hypotheses was appreciated by
Hirsch a hundred years ago, though the data available at
that time were so limited that he devoted to it only 14 of
the 2,000 pages of his great work on geographical and
historical pathology. It is notable, moreover, that study
of the two cancers which Hirsch regarded as having a clearly
defined geographical demarcation – the sweeps' cancer of
the scrotum in England and the Kangri cancer of the skin
of the abdomen in Kashmir – has since provided much
valuable information about the causes of cancer in general.

Until recently, investigation of the subject was limited
to a few countries which were able to provide high quality
mortality data, and to a handful of districts in which attempts
had been made to register all the locally occurring cancers.
In other parts of the world, indeed in the greater part of
it, the only useful data were hospital or autopsy series, and
these provided very biased estimates of the relative frequency of different types of cancer and no record of their
actual incidence. Otherwise there was no information at all.
The principal difficulty was, therefore, lack of data.

Today, the amount of data available for study has increased
enormously; and although there are still wide areas for
which information is scanty, we are beginning to be able to
draw a cancer map that spreads over all continents and

leaves relatively few countries completely blank. The great difficulty now is not so much lack of data as knowing whether the data are comparable.

The first problem we have to face in a study of this kind is the difficulty caused by differences in the age distribution of the different populations; cancer incidence varies so greatly with age (the incidence of some types increasing five hundred times over a span of fifty years) that differences in the proportion of the population in the various age groups can produce differences in the crude cancer incidence rates as great as those produced by differences in the prevalence of carcinogenic factors. The second problem is that not all data are equally reliable; the value of mortality data depends on the accuracy of death certification, which in turn depends on the quality and accessibility of the medical services. The diagnoses are not so often in question where incidence data are concerned because these are not usually collected unless the population is provided with a fairly high standard of medical service; but they can be grossly misleading if a proportion of the population fails to make use of the services, or if registration of diagnosed cases is incomplete.

The problem introduced by differences in age distribution can be partly overcome by the use of rates standardized for age, and this would be an adequate solution if cancer incidence varied with age in the same way in all countries. Unfortunately it does not. In some areas the recorded incidence fails to increase progressively with age, either because of under diagnosis in old age, or because of biases in the reporting of ages, or because of real differences in the age distribution of the disease; and a comparison of standardized rates leads to different conclusions, depending on the age distribution of the standard population. Ideally, comparisons should be made between rates for individual five-year age groups. This, however, is seldom practicable: first because the numbers of cases recorded in incidence studies are often small, so that the rates would be liable to large random fluctuations; and secondly because the number of rates that would have to be examined is so large, and the results of comparisons at different ages so variable, that it would be extremely difficult to digest all the material and obtain a general picture of the situation.

In these circumstances, the best that can be done is to limit the comparisons between areas to a narrow range in which cancer is fairly frequent but which excludes ages where the decreased reliability of the rates is likely to be a major factor. For the principal cancers of adult life comparison has, therefore, been limited to ages 35 to 64 years and within these limits the rates have been standardized for age, using as the standard the average world population which was suggested by Mitsuo Segi. This limitation has the advantage that it also eliminates the age groups in which the utilization of medical services is likely to be least complete, and it reduces the effect of differences in the social environment which may have been in part responsible for the current incidence of cancer but which have long since disappeared (Doll and Cook, 1967).

Geographical distribution

Figures that can be used for geographical comparisons may be obtained from special studies of cancer incidence, from national mortality statistics and, in a few special cases, from clinical and pathological records. Incidence data are now available for some fifty different populations; some have been collected by national or regional cancer registries, such as the *Danish National Cancer Registry* and the *South Metropolitan Cancer Registry* in England, some obtained as a result of a special investigation carried out over a few years in a selected area, such as Higginson and Oettlé's study of Africans in Johannesburg, and Correa and Llanos' study of Cali, Colombia. Not all the data are sufficiently complete for the present purpose and, for the most part, comparisons are confined to those accepted by a Committee of the *International Union against Cancer* for inclusion in a book dealing with cancer incidence throughout the world (Doll, Payne & Waterhouse, 1966).

Mortality statistics for the main types of cancer have been published for forty-eight countries and for the urban areas of the fifteen Soviet republics (World Health Organization, 1966; Segi and Kurihara, 1964; Merkova, Trerkovnogo and Kaufman, 1963). The value of the figures is, however, very variable and with few exceptions I have felt justified in using only those from Europe, North America, Australasia and Soviet Asia. To make mortality comparable with incidence data, it has been necessary to multiply the mortality rates by a factor to allow for some cancers being cured and for others, though still present, not being regarded as the cause of death. Fortunately incidence and mortality rates for the same periods are available in eight countries, and this allows estimates to be made of the appropriate factor for each type of cancer. The factors, and the mortality rates to which they have been applied, will be listed elsewhere (Doll, 1967).

Finally, there is an immense choice of clinical and pathological records. Few of these can be used to provide a useful estimate of incidence, but in exceptional cases such records may provide clear evidence of a situation that is qualitatively different from that found in other parts of the world. They are particularly useful in relation to such cancers as Burkitt's lymphoma, Kaposi's sarcoma and primary carcinoma of the liver and I have occasionally used selected records relating to these cancers for this purpose.

The distribution of five of the principal adult cancers is shown diagramatically in the appendix in plates I to V. Plate I shows the distribution of cancer of the oesophagus in men. Three foci of very high incidence are shown – in the Ghurjev region of Kazakhstan on the north coast of the Caspian, among Africans in the Transkei region of Cape Province, and among Africans in Bulawayo. Areas of very high incidence are also known to exist in the north of Honan province in China and in Curaçao, but they are not illustrated because comparable figures are not available. In all these areas cancer of the oesophagus is the commonest cancer in men. In the Ghurjev region, where the rate is highest, cancer of the oesophagus is two hundred times as common as in Holland or Nigeria, and about three times as common as lung cancer is in London. One notable feature of the Transkei focus is that the disease has appeared in the memory of doctors who are still practising; in a hospital with two hundred beds, one or two cases are admitted each week. The epidemic is apparently spreading to some other South African populations and is now beginning to attain considerable proportions among the Cape Coloured in Cape Town.

Whenever special studies have been made a relationship has always been found with both smoking and alcohol consumption, and this holds whether the incidence is low, as in England, Sweden and the United States, moderate, as in India and France, or high, as in the Transkei. It is clear, however, that these factors alone do not produce much disease and they certainly cannot account for the very high incidence recorded in some parts of the world. An exception may be France, where the association with alcohol consumption is particularly close, but it is not clear why the rate should be so much higher there than in other countries where large amounts of alcohol are consumed. Burrell, Roach and Shadwell have recently suggested that local soil deficiencies may result in diseased and infected crops in the Transkei and that these, possibly by the production of nitrosamines, may be responsible for the disease. The evidence is not convincing, however, and the hypothesis fails to account for the recent spread of the disease to the Cape Coloured.

Plate II shows the distribution of cancer of the stomach. High rates are more common than with cancer of the oesophagus, but the highest rates never equal that for cancer of the oesophagus in the Ghurjev district and the lowest rates are never as low as those for cancer of the oesophagus in Holland, Nigeria, or Canada. The range is, therefore, only about thirty-fold from Russia and Japan to Uganda and Mozambique. The most striking feature of the map is the gradient of incidence across Europe from Russia to south-western England and further across the Atlantic to the white population of the United States. Outside eastern Europe, high or very high rates are found in Japan, Iceland

and Chile. In India, exemplified by the figures for Bombay, the rate is similar to that in Connecticut. In most parts of Africa the rate is low; but there is almost certainly a focus of moderately high incidence in the Kivu district of the Congo, where cancer of the stomach is the commonest cancer in men, and there may also be some high incidence areas in Tanzania.

Genetic factors clearly play some part in the production of the disease, since in high and low incidence areas alike people belonging to blood group A have 20 per cent more gastric cancer than people belonging to the other blood groups; but it is equally clear that they are not responsible for the big differences recorded between areas, which cut across racial lines. The non-white population of the United States has, for example, more gastric cancer than the white, whereas all European populations have more than the negro populations in Africa. It is notable also that the Japanese in Hawaii have a rate which resembles that of their host culture more closely than that of their homeland.

One encouraging feature is that the incidence of gastric cancer is falling. Mortality rates show a sharp fall nearly everywhere, except in Japan; and nowhere is the rate of fall faster than in the United States where there has been a 40 per cent drop in mortality spread fairly evenly over all ages, in twelve years, a fall which certainly cannot be attributed to improvement in treatment. The American rate for whites is now, in fact, the lowest anywhere in the world outside some of the relatively undeveloped areas of Africa.

Assuredly carcinogenic factors must be present in some

simple diets – for instance in that of the poorer classes in Japan which has largely consisted of rice, and in the diet of fish, mutton and potatoes which was staple in Iceland before the war. This has suggested that a dietary deficiency may be responsible for the disease. Equally clearly the elaborate methods of food processing in the United States have apparently not yet introduced any factors carcinogenic to the human stomach and it is pleasant to note that large amounts of charcoal grilled steak, with their concomitant content of 3–4: benzpyrene, do not appear to be harmful under American conditions. The evidence of a relationship with smoked fish (Dungal, 1961) is unconvincing, and alcohol and tobacco have, for this type of cancer, been unequivocally exculpated. It is perhaps possible that some carcinogenic factors can be produced by the deterioration of food on storage: if this is so, the low rate of gastric cancer in the United States could be attributed to improved methods of food preservation; but it would have to be a type of deterioration that could take place on prolonged storage in a cold climate.

Plate III shows the distribution of cancer of the lung. The range of variation is somewhat greater than for cancer of the stomach, the incidence varying forty-fold between Britain and parts of Africa. Contrary to what is sometimes said, cancer of the lung is quite common in eastern Europe and in the towns of the Soviet Union. It is notable, however, that it is higher in Britain than in other Anglo-Saxon communities, particularly Australia and Canada where the incidence at ages 35–64 years is about 60 per cent lower than in Britain.

Wherever the disease is now common it has become so

only in the last thirty or forty years. In Britain, where the increase has been most marked, the male mortality at ages 35 to 64 years, standardized for age, increased twenty-fold between 1923 and 1964. In all countries the increase has been more marked in men than in women, but the trend in the sex ratio has been reversed in Britain for the last eight years, the rate of increase becoming greater in women than in men.

There is now much evidence to suggest that this widespread increase in incidence is due to an increase in cigarette smoking. The mortality from lung cancer among British doctors, for example, is forty times greater in men smoking thirty-five or more cigarettes a day than in life-long non-smokers (Doll and Hill, 1964) and between these two extremes the mortality increases in proportion to the amount smoked. Similar observations in other countries lead to the same general conclusion, but it is notable that the increase in mortality per unit amount smoked is usually less. As a result the incidence is lower in several countries even though the average consumption of cigarettes per head is higher.

One possible explanation of this discrepancy would be that cigarette smoking exerts a greater effect on tissue that has been prepared by some other agent, for example, by atmospheric pollution. Some of the recorded differences can, however, be attributed to differences in the history of past cigarette consumption, and much of the rest may be due to differences in the way cigarettes are smoked, and perhaps also to the type of tobacco used. The length of butt discarded in different countries is known to vary and Wynder and Fairchild have found that the average number of puffs taken per cigarette varies substantially between New York and London. Evidently it cannot be assumed that smoking the same number of cigarettes a day provides the same degree of exposure to carcinogenic agents in all countries and in all social milieux.

Plate IV shows the distribution of cancer of the colon. The maximum incidence is a quarter of that for cancer of the lung and the range is only ten-fold. Figures have not been reported for so many countries – there is a relative lack of data for eastern Europe in particular – and presumably this implies that the disease is generally less frequent in those countries. The most noteworthy feature of the map is that the highest rates are almost always reported for populations with Anglo-American cultures; in fact, Uruguay is the only non-Anglo-American country to appear in the first ten. For this type of cancer, differences in incidence are clearly related to culture and not to race. In the United States the disease is almost equally common in whites and none-whites, and in Hawaii it is equally common among Caucasians, Japanese and Hawaiians. In contrast, it is rare among Africans everywhere in Africa and among the Japanese in Japan. Clinical series show that the ratio of the numbers of cancers in the right and left half of the colon also varies; the proportion of right-sided cancers is higher when the disease is rare, so that the range of variation must be greater for cancer of the sigmoid colon than for cancer of the caecum.

Plate V shows the distribution of cancer of the breast in women. Here the most notable feature is the steady reduction in incidence from west to east – from Canada and the United States across the Atlantic to western, central and eastern Europe, and finally to central Asia; this gradient, it may be noted, is exactly the reverse of that found with cancer of the stomach. Low rates are also found in Taiwan, Uganda and Mozambique, but no very low rates are found anywhere.

Within countries, cancer of the breast tends to run in families, but genetic factors cannot account for the principal geographical differences. Non-whites, for examples, have the same rate as whites in the United States, although the disease is rare among Africans in Africa, and the Japanese in Hawaii suffer a rate which is appreciably higher than that of the Japanese in Japan. Fertility and prolonged lactation are associated with lower rates, and may have a minor protective effect. Such factors, however, are inadequate to account for the eight-fold differences between communities. The very striking gradient from west to east across Europe suggests the possibility that a dietetic factor may play a part.

Plate VI shows the distribution of cancer of the liver in men, but for ages 15 to 44 years instead of ages 35 to 64 years. A different scale has therefore been used and the various colours represent rates equal to one-eighth of those shown previously. This age group has been chosen partly because liver cancer appears early in adult life in countries where it is common, and partly to reduce confusion between primary and secondary liver cancer, and between liver cancer and cancer of the large bile ducts, a confusion that becomes increasingly difficult to avoid at older ages, when gastric, colonic, pulmonary and gall bladder cancers are all relatively frequent.

In young adult life, liver cancer is rare everywhere except in the tropics; but it is not uniformly common in the tropics, and varies enormously from place to place. In Lourenço Marques, Mozambique, it is as common as lung cancer is in England among men twenty years older, and it is a thousand times as common as primary liver cancer in most of Europe; in contrast, it is no commoner in Puerto Rico than in the United States. Hospital series show that it occurs fairly widely throughout East and West Africa; but the frequency does not approach that reported from Mozambique anywhere except, perhaps, in Senegal and some other parts of the West African coast. Hospital series show that it is common in Hong Kong and probably also in much of South China. The suggestion that it may be due to aflatoxin formed in ground nuts and cereals stored under hot and humid conditions is attractive, but there is no reason to suppose that aflatoxin is that much more prevalent in Mozambique than elsewhere. The disease cannot be related to liver damage due to kwashiorkor in infancy, nor does it appear to have any simple relation to the frequency of viral hepatitis.

The data available for most cancers other than those discussed above are relatively incomplete. Few countries publish mortality rates in as much detail as the Registrars General of Great Britain, and many limit themselves to the commonest diseases and the broad categories in the World Health Organization's abridged lists of causes of death. Mortality rates, moreover, provide only a poor indication of incidence for curable cancers like those of the lip and skin, or for cancers like sarcoma of bone, which tend to be confused with other and secondary cancers in the classification of causes of death. For these, our knowledge is limited to that obtained from cancer registries, special surveys of incidence, and hospital and pathological records. The results of some such studies are summarized in Table 1; unless otherwise stated, the rates all refer to men aged 35 to 64 years. High rates based on fewer than fifteen cases have been ignored and those based on fifteen to twenty-nine

TABLE I

Variation in Cancer Incidence*

Range of rates (high divided by low)	Type of primary cancer	High incidence areas	Low incidence areas
1,000	liver (ages 15–44 years)	Lourenço Marques	Alberta, Saskatchewan Norway, Sweden N.Y. State, Birmingham region
200	oesophagus	Ghurjev district of Kazakhstan	Alberta, Manitoba, Netherlands, Ibadan
100	penis	Kingston (Jamaica) *Uganda*	Israel
100	nasopharynx	Chinese (Singapore)	Uganda Cali (Colombia) Chile, Finland
50	lip	Saskatchewan, Alberta, New Brunswick	Lourenço Marques Uganda Hawaii (Japanese, Hawaiians) Japan Johannesburg (Africans)

* Men aged 35 to 64 years, unless specified otherwise.

TABLE 1—*continued*

Range of rates (high divided by low)	Type of primary cancer	High incidence areas	Low incidence areas
40	skin	New Brunswick, Saskatchewan, Alberta, Cali (Colombia)	Johannesburg (Africans) Ibadan
40	bronchus	Liverpool, Birmingham	Uganda Ibadan
30	stomach	Japan Iceland	Lourenço Marques Uganda
30	chorion-epithelioma (♀ ages 15–44 years)	*Ibadan* *Japan*	Iceland, Hawaii Alberta, Manitoba, Newfoundland, Connecticut, Birmingham region Denmark
30	pharynx	Puerto Rico	Ibadan, Johannesburg (Africans) Iceland, Japan
20	mouth	Bombay	Uganda, Hawaii (Hawaiians) Iceland, Denmark, Chile
20	corpus uteri (♀)	Saskatchewan Hawaii (Caucasians)	Ibadan, Johannesburg (Africans) Lourenço Marques Uganda
20	cervix uteri (♀)	Puerto Ricans (New York) Cali (Colombia) Johannesburg (Africans) Hawaii (Hawaiians)	Jewesses (New York) Israel South Metropolitan region (England) Birmingham region

TABLE I—*continued*

Range of rates (high divided by low)	Type of primary cancer	High incidence areas	Low incidence areas
10–15	rectum	Denmark, New Zealand	Lourenço Marques, Johannesburg (Africans) Ibadan
10–15	thyroid	*Cali (Colombia)* Hawaii (all groups combined)	Uganda, Johannesburg (Africans) Liverpool, Southwestern England
10	tongue	Puerto Rico	Lourenço Marques, Uganda, Alberta, Japan, Israel
10	colon	Connecticut New Zealand	Uganda, Ibadan, Johannesburg (Africans)
10	testis	Denmark, New Zealand	Ibadan, Uganda, Johannesburg (Africans) Kingston (Jamaica) Japan
10	kidney	Iceland, Sweden	Ibadan, Uganda, Japan
10	melanoma	New Zealand, Connecticut, Norway	Hawaii (Japanese, Hawaiians) Japan Iceland, Ibadan, Johannesburg (Africans)

cases are shown in italics. Zero rates have been ignored in calculating the range, and areas in which no cases were reported are shown as low rates only if a low rate was reported for other similar populations.

For cancer arising in the salivary glands, gall bladder and major bile ducts, pancreas, nasal sinuses, larynx, breast, ovary, prostate, bladder, bone, and connective tissue, and for lympho- and reticulosarcoma, Hodgkin's disease and multiple myelomatosis, the range of variation appears to be between three- and ten-fold. Greater differences are recorded for some types, but the cancers are rare and some of the populations are small, so that the figures are liable to substantial random error. Only leukaemia seems likely to vary less than three-fold. In young adult life the rates are particularly stable, and it may well be that in this age group the true incidence of leukaemia does not vary by more than a factor of two.

As new areas are studied and more information is obtained even greater variations are likely to be observed, particularly if it also becomes possible to separate the various types of cancer that occur in each site: much more striking results might be obtained if, for example, it was possible to separate the figures for seminoma and teratoma of the testis and for myeloid and lymphatic leukaemia. To achieve this for all cancers on a large scale, is a task of such magnitude that it is unlikely to be completed for many years, by which time some of the most revealing differences may have been eliminated by the spread of a uniform culture. Meanwhile, however, we can obtain some rough but useful estimates from clinical and pathological records and the calculation of the proportions which particular cancers contribute to the total. When, nearly ninety years ago, Maxwell reported that twenty-seven of the fifty-four cancer cases seen at the Kashmir Mission Dispensary were epitheliomas of the abdominal wall and seventeen were tumors of the skin of the thigh, no one could doubt that the people of the vale of Kashmir were exposed to some special risk of developing cancer at these unusual sites. Nor, now, can there be any doubt that the inhabitants of central Africa have a special risk of developing Kaposi's sarcoma, when this disease accounts for 10 per cent of all cancers in pathological series from this area; nor that a local factor is responsible for Burkitt's lymphoma when it accounts for half of all the childhood cancers diagnosed in Kampala.

Temporal distribution

Changes in the incidence of cancer with time are more difficult to establish than changes from place to place, for while it is theoretically possible to check observations in different areas by a planned study, using comparable methods in each area, it is impossible to recall a time that is past and we have no alternative but to make do, as well as we can, with the material that is already to hand. This difficult situation is intensified by the fact that with few exceptions incidence data have been collected for only a short time and we have to rely on the indirect evidence of mortality. Moreover, the accuracy of medical diagnosis, the provision of medical services, and the efficacy of treatment have everywhere been steadily improved. In these circumstances it is not surprising that speculations about changes in incidence have always been hotly debated and that few confident conclusions are possible.

Three important changes in cancer incidence have already been referred to – the widespread increase in cancer of the lung, the increase of cancer of the oesophagus in the Transkei, and the widespread reduction in cancer of the stomach – and there can be little serious doubt that these have all been real. For other cancers the evidence is more difficult to interpret. Segi and Kurihara's study of cancer mortality in twenty-four countries shows that, so far as mortality is concerned, change is the rule and stability the exception. Over the last fifteen years the mortality from leukaemia and from cancers of the pancreas and urogenital tract has increased nearly everywhere – the first two types in both sexes, the last mainly in men. Other cancers that appear to have become more common include cancers of the breast, ovary and prostate, but the trend has not been the same everywhere and in some countries the death rate has been steady. Opposite trends have been shown by cancers of the uterus (cervix and body combined) and by cancers of the mouth, pharynx and oesophagus in men. These last three types of cancer have, however, shown an increasing mortality in France and in Italy. For other cancers, including cancers of the intestine, rectum and larynx, no general rule can be discerned; in some countries the death rates have gone up, in others down.

Comparisons can be made over longer periods in a few countries, but they become more hazardous as the length of the period increases. As with geographical comparisons their validity can be improved by excluding the oldest age groups and the comparisons are probably best made only over the age range of 35 to 64 years.

Changes in the death rate for different types of cancer in England and Wales over a forty-year period are shown in Table 2. The increase in the mortality from lung cancer is clearly of a different order of magnitude from that recorded for any other type. The others for which an increase in mortality has been recorded are all cancers of 'inaccessible' sites and improved methods of diagnosis must be presumed

TABLE 2

Changes in cancer mortality in England and Wales, 1921–25 to 1964 (ages 35–64 years, standardized for age*)

Type of primary cancer	1964 rate as per cent of rate in 1921–25
lung	2188
leukaemia	320
kidney	205
ovaries (♀) pancreas Hodgkin's disease bladder	150–199
testis breast (♀) prostate	80–124
stomach intestines skin rectum	50–79
uterus (♀) pharynx vulva & vagina (♀) oesophagus	33–49
larynx penis & scrotum	25–32
mouth + tonsil	11
lip tongue	7

* Men unless specified otherwise.

to have contributed a part. Some of the increases may well be real, however, and in the case of leukaemia it has been argued that this is particularly likely to be true for the myeloid types (Court Brown, Doll and Hill, 1964). Improved treatment is likely to have contributed to the reduction in mortality from cancer of the intestines, rectum, and larynx, but it can hardly have been responsible for the drop in the death rate from cancer of the oseophagus, nor for the very large drop in the mortality from cancers of the mouth, lip and tongue. Further information, that is helpful in interpreting the trends, can be obtained by comparing the age-specific mortality of cohorts born at different periods (Case, 1956). In this way it has been possible to show that the unusual shape of the curve relating mortality to age in cancer of the lung is readily explained by increasing exposure of different cohorts to an environmental carcinogen.

Space-time clusters

As well as varying in time and in space the incidence of a disease may vary in both dimensions together; indeed all cancers that vary in space are probably also varying in time, but the rate of variation in time is usually so slow that it is not easily recognized. For many of these diseases the fact that cases cluster in both dimensions in a related way adds little or nothing to the observation that they vary in each separately. In some circumstances, however, the recognition of space-time clustering may provide important new evidence which would not easily be obtained from separate studies of the geographical and temporal distribution of the disease. Consider the common cold. It occurs almost equally in all parts of the country and every year, and examination of its incidence in different towns and in different years provides little information of aetiological interest. When, however, observations are made on individuals, it is obvious that colds spread from one member of a family to another and that having passed through a household they often do not occur in the same family again for several months. This type of behaviour is typical of endemic infectious diseases and it is usually easy to recognize. It is, however, difficult to recognize if the disease is rare or if the majority of infected people show only minor and atypical symptoms or no symptoms at all. The infectious nature of endemic poliomyelitis in tropical countries was, for example, overlooked until its characteristics were worked out in temperate climates where infection was normally less common and the disease occurred in waves at intervals of several years.

When a disease is endemic and extremely rare, the appearance of three or four cases in a small area within a short time attracts attention and creates the appearance of a small epidemic. Such 'epidemics' are, however, bound to occur from time to time by chance alone and, in these circumstances, it may be extremely difficult to decide whether the amount of clustering that has been observed is more than can reasonably be attributed to chance, or whether it provides *a priori* evidence of the temporary appearance of a causative agent.

Until recently it has not been possible to measure with any accuracy the probability that a series of clusters might be due to chance. The problem was solved, however, in essence when Knox pointed out that all that needed to be done was to measure the distance between pairs of cases in time and in space, and to see whether those pairs that occurred close together in time also tended to be close together in space. His method, or others derived from it, has been applied to two types of cancer that have been suspected of having an infectious origin – childhood leukaemia and Burkitt's lymphoma.

Knox originally studied childhood leukaemia in Northumberland and Durham over a ten-year period and he found that among ninety-six children with lymphoblastic leukaemia which first appeared under the age of six years, there were five pairs who lived within one kilometre of each other and who developed the disease within a period of sixty days. This degree of clustering would have occurred by chance only once in five hundred times, and it provided good grounds for suggesting that the disease might occur in small epidemics. It could not, however, be regarded as proof of a real tendency for clustering, as there had been no previous reason to select this special subgroup of affected children, nor to limit the space and time differences to one kilometre and sixty days. Indeed, no clustering was found among cases that occurred in older children or were of other cytological types. Subsequent studies have provided conflicting results. Some have indicated less marked clustering within wider limits, and a study of four hundred and eighty-three cases of childhood leukaemias in Greater London over a ten-year period failed to provide any evidence of clustering at all. So far as they go, therefore, these epidemiological studies cannot be regarded as providing any real support for the concept that childhood leukaemia is due to an infectious agent.

The results obtained with Burkitt's lymphoma provide a
marked contrast. Pike, Williams and Wright examined
the distribution of cases in one district of Uganda over a
six-year period and showed that the disease spread from
one part of the district to another and then back again in
a way that was almost impossible to attribute to chance*.
Moreover, the division into time intervals could be made
objectively and the evidence is self-contained and does not
depend on repetition in a further set of data. The interpretation of these results is, however, open to question.
They could be due to a similar space-time clustering of the
population (as, for example, when a large body of pilgrims
visits a holy place over a religious festival); but no one who
worked in the area believed that this type of population
movement had occurred. Alternatively they might be due
to a similar movement of diagnostic interest, as, for
example, could happen in the trail of one of Mr. Burkitt's
safaris; this, however, is unlikely as the area had been
chosen because it contained only three hospitals, and the
doctors in these hospitals had been interested in the
disease since before the period began. Finally, they might
be due to the movements of the causative agent. As Dr.
Pike has pointed out, this need not be a living organism –
an inadequately protected mobile X-ray mass radiography
unit might leave a trail of cases of leukaemia behind it –
butn on-infectious agents that could behave like this are
difficult to envisage. In fact, the evidence accords well
with the picture of Burkitt's lymphoma as being due to a
virus to which all are exposed, but which produces overt
cancer in only a small minority of cases.

* At the highest estimate $P = \cdot 005$.

Chapter 4

AETIOLOGICAL FACTORS

Scope of review

The number of substances that are known to cause cancer is now so large, and the substances themselves so widespread that, as Maurice Goldblatt said, it is a lucky man who succeeds in getting out of this world alive! Many of these substances, however, have been identified by animal experiments and it does not necessarily follow that a substance which causes cancer in a mouse or a guinea pig will cause a cancer in man; nor does it follow that, because it causes a cancer on subcutaneous injection, it will also cause one when ingested or brought into contact with the skin. The fact that a substance has been shown to be carcinogenic under experimental conditions is, however, of considerable value when we are interpreting the results of observations on man – particularly if the result has been reproduced in several different species. In this situation, the observation of an unusually high incidence of cancer in a group of men exposed to the substance in the same way as experimental animals are exposed, is sufficient to justify us in assuming that the substance is responsible for the human tumours, and attempting to prevent the disease by reducing the exposure.

In other circumstances, when action depends on human observations alone, the chain of reasoning must be more nearly complete, and every possible alternative explanation should be considered. The exact stage at which it becomes reasonable to try a prophylactic experiment will depend upon a careful balancing of the extent of the risk against the degree of ease with which the suspected agent may be removed and the possible consequences of removing it.

In the present chapter, I make no attempt to review the relevant animal experiments, but confine myself to information obtained from observations on man. Much of it is well known, and in this case I shall merely summarize the conclusions, reserving for more detailed review evidence that is relatively new or is open to different interpretations.

For convenience, I shall consider the evidence under five heads – relating to carcinogenic factors that occur generally, or locally, are dependent on the behaviour of the individual, are introduced by medical investigation or treatment, or are related to the occurrence of other diseases.

Genetic factors will be considered separately in chapter 6.

General environment

Conclusive evidence that *ionizing radiations* can cause cancer is provided by a wide range of observations on man and experiments with animals. Many types of cancer have been produced, and the evidence is so extensive that it is reasonable to assume that all tissues, or nearly all, are susceptible. Observations include the high incidence of carcinoma of the skin of the hand among the early radiologists, carcinoma of the lung among men who were exposed to high concentrations of radon in the mines of Schneeberg and Jachymov, in the uranium mines of Colorado, or the fluorspar mines of Newfoundland; bone sarcoma among women employed as luminizers in the United States; leukaemia and, to a lesser extent, other cancers among the survivors of the atomic explosions in Hiroshima and

Nagasaki; leukaemia and other cancers in exposed sites among patients irradiated for ankylosing spondylitis; leukaemia and carcinoma of the thyroid among children irradiated at birth for a putatively enlarged thymus; all the common childhood cancers among children irradiated in utero; and reticulo-endothelioma of the liver in patients injected with thorotrast. In addition many individual cancers have been observed in a wide range of tissues that had been seriously damaged by exposure to large amounts of radiation.

In most of these examples the doses of radiation have been large, and it does not follow that an effect is produced by the small doses received from radon in the air, from radio-active substances in land, buildings, and our own bodies, and from cosmic rays. Not only is the amount of radiation received from these sources (approximately 0·1 rad per year) very small, but it is received at about one hundred millionth of the rate at which diagnostic and therapeutic X-rays are given. If recovery from the type of damage that induced cancer is possible, this low rate may substantially modify the response of the tissues. Direct observation of the effect produced by such small doses – as, for example, is theoretically possible in Aberdeen where background radiation is increased by 20 per cent by the widespread use of granite as a building material – is quite impracticable, because of the multiplicity of other factors that affect cancer incidence; and we have to rely on the indirect approach of extrapolation from the effect of the very much higher doses that can be estimated quantitatively.

The method of extrapolation that has been used by the International Commission on Radiological Protection (1966), is to assume a linear relationship between dose of radiation and incidence of the induced effect. This procedure, as the United Nations Scientific Committee on the Effects of Atomic Radiation (1964) concluded, is likely to indicate an upper limit of risk because 'it is unlikely that the risk per unit dose at very low doses will be any greater than at high doses and is likely to be much less.' More reliable estimates can, however, be made only when we have a full understanding of the biological mechanisms by which the effects are produced, and can make adequate allowance for the extension of the extrapolation to levels of irradiation which are several orders of magnitude smaller than those that have produced the observed results. The evidence for the use of a linear relationship rather than any other is discussed in chapter 5.

From the available data, the International Commission concluded that exposure of the whole body to one rad per year might lead to an annual rate of twenty cases of leukaemia per million persons and that the incidence of other fatal neoplasms would be approximately the same. Since the mortality from all neoplasms in England and Wales is approximately 2,000 per million persons per year, background radiation (amounting to 0·1 rad per year) is clearly unlikely to account for more than a negligible proportion of all cancers. For leukaemia the position is somewhat different. At ages 15 to 44 years the mean annual death rate is approximately 20 to 24 per million per year, so that at these ages the contribution of background radiation may be of the order of 10 per cent. It is possible also that background radiation may be responsible for a similar proportion of some of the less common cancers – particularly perhaps for sarcoma of bone. There is nothing in the very limited quantitative data that have yet been collected for bone tumours in luminizers that would rule out the possibility that the natural body burden of radium (approximately 0·0001μc) could cause a substantial proportion of the normal death rate from bone tumours which, in England and Wales, ranges from one to 14 per million persons per year at different ages.

Another type of radiation that is known to be carcinogenic is the sun's *ultraviolet radiation* in the range of 2,900 to 3,300 Angström units. In large amounts these rays are carcinogenic to the skin of animals, but the order of dose that man receives in the course of his normal daily – or in Britain perhaps monthly – exposure, appears also to be responsible for a large proportion of cancers of the skin and lip.

The theory that sunlight is a primary cause of skin cancer was accepted by dermatologists more than fifty years ago, at which time the evidence was entirely clinical and epidemiological. It had been observed that: (i) cancers of the skin were found most frequently on those parts of the body that were habitually exposed to sunlight; (ii) the incidence was greater in those parts of the world which received the greatest amount of sunlight; (iii) the condition was commoner in outdoor workers than indoor; and (iv) it was more prevalent in light skinned people than in dark.

More recent evidence has strengthened these conclusions, and practically all cancers of the skin of the face can now be attributed to this cause. Dorn and Cutler, for example, showed that the incidence in white people in the United

States increased steadily as latitude decreased, and Blum showed that the change in incidence parallelled fairly closely the change in the amount of ultraviolet light received at the earth's surface. Little corresponding change takes place in negroes, and it is now clear that most cancers of the skin in negroes are a different form of the disease with different causes. Rodent ulcer is rare in negroes, and most cases of skin cancer occur on the limbs, particularly, in Africa, in long-standing 'tropical ulcers' on the legs (see p. 87).

Essentially the same type of evidence implicates sunlight as a cause of cancer of the lip; but the quantitative relationship is less clear because lip cancer is also related to smoking (see p. 79).

Local environment

Of the many local factors that could be a cause of cancer the most interesting and potentially the most important is *pollution of the atmosphere* with chimney smoke and the exhaust fumes of motor vehicles. These smokes and fumes contain substantial quantities of 3:4-benzpyrene and other polycyclic hydrocarbons that are carcinogenic to animals; they come into direct contact with the bronchial mucosa in normal respiration; they contaminate the skin and reach the gastro-intestinal tract by contaminating food; and, in the case of exhaust fumes, the amount liberated on the roads has increased enormously in the last fifty years, and will in all probability continue to do so in the next.

At first sight, atmospheric pollution might well be regarded as a major cause of lung cancer – which has also increased enormously in incidence and has everywhere been found to be commoner in towns than in the countryside. Indeed, when the Medical Research Council began its inquiry into the aetiology of the disease in 1947, coal smoke and motor fumes headed the list of factors to be studied (Doll and Hill, 1950). Unfortunately neither this inquiry nor any subsequent ones have been able to provide a decisive answer, and it is extremely difficult to conceive of any epidemiological study that would.

Two difficulties complicate investigation: first, exposure to atmospheric pollution is something that people share in common, and though we can pick out groups of people who have had more or less exposure, it is difficult to measure the exposure of an individual and to make any quantitative estimates of the difference in the extent to which different people have been personally exposed. Secondly, pollution is a product of life in towns and it is difficult to separate its effect from that of other factors which accompany urban residence, including smoking habits, respiratory infection, and more readily available diagnostic facilities. What has become clear is that atmospheric pollution cannot be the sole, or even the most important, cause of lung cancer. Large prospective studies in this country and the United States agree in showing that the mortality rate among non-smokers is extremely small, irrespective of where the non-smokers have lived. It is difficult to make a precise estimate of the rates from different parts of the country because of the very small number of cases of lung cancer among non-smokers that have been observed. If, however, we take the retrospective studies into account also — and it is remarkable how similar the results of the two methods of enquiry have been — it seems reasonable to conclude

that the rate among men living in the biggest cities is two
to three times that of men living in rural areas, whereas
within each area the rate among cigarette smokers is
about ten times that among non-smokers.

Within each area the incidence (or mortality) increases
with amount smoked, but the rate nearly always remains
higher in the big cities and the ratio of the rates at each
level of smoking remains approximately the same (except
sometimes in the heaviest smoking categories when the
difference may disappear).

It would seem possible, therefore, that pollution – or
some other factor associated with the circumstances of urban
life – acts synergistically with cigarette smoking, and by so
doing may contribute to up to 50 per cent of the total
lung cancer mortality.

Further evidence which tends to support this possibility
comes from examination of the incidence of lung cancer in
the locally-born inhabitants of Australia, New Zealand,
South Africa and the United States in comparison with
that in immigrants from Britain.

In each case the incidence of lung cancer in the immigrants is higher – and sometimes substantially higher. This
cannot be explained by differences in current cigarette consumption, and it appears as if the British immigrants
have brought with them a risk due to damage done years
before in their homeland.

The evidence is, however, not all readily explicable on
this hypothesis. Haenszel, Loveland, and Sirken, for example,
found that even within the United States the incidence
appeared to be higher in men who had migrated from rural
areas into large towns than in men who had lived all their

life in the cities – suggesting that the increased risk might be in some way associated with the character of a migrant rather than with the place he had come from. And Buck and Brown, who undertook a large-scale study of the mortality from lung cancer and chronic bronchitis in England on behalf of the Tobacco Research Council, found that the incidence of lung cancer correlated with the density of population of a town, and not independently with any measured element of the pollution in its air. This last finding was particularly impressive because it contrasted with the findings on chronic bronchitis, the incidence of which correlated well with both the smoke and the SO_2 content of town air.

Two other points have also to be borne in mind. First, the diagnosis of lung cancer is still not always accurate and relatively more cases may be missed in rural areas where facilities are less readily available. Secondly, the sort of differences in smoking habits that were mentioned earlier in relation to the geographical distribution of lung cancer (p. 38) may also play a part. When one factor can be responsible for a forty-fold difference in incidence (as the amount of cigarette smoking can be), it is as well to proceed cautiously before asserting that a two-fold difference persists after this factor has been allowed for.

Perhaps the most useful piece of evidence is that derived from a study of the mortality of *gasworkers* – men who, in the course of their daily work, are exposed to large quantities of tar fumes similar in character to the tar which urban dwellers inspire in town air. Lawther, Commins, and Waller examined air in the retort houses of some typical gasworks and found extreme concentrations of 3:4-

benzpyrene that were ten thousand times as great as the average amount in the air of London. Such concentrations were, of course, seldom if ever breathed, but the average concentration inspired throughout a shift appeared to be about a hundred times the London average. As the mortality from lung cancer among the retort house workers was less than double that of gasfitters who worked in the streets and houses of the town (the actual difference was 70 per cent), two things would appear to follow. First, coal tar can, in suitable circumstances, cause lung cancer. Secondly, the amount of polycyclic hydrocarbons in town air is much too small to double the incidence of lung cancer among cigarette smokers.

No final conclusion about the effect of urban atmospheric pollution is yet possible. On present evidence one can assess it only within very wide limits. At the most it may contribute to 50 per cent of all lung cancer, at the least to 0 per cent; and the best estimate probably lies much nearer the latter figure than the former.

Another 'local' factor which has recently become prominent is *asbestos*. That this can cause two types of cancer – the normal bronchial carcinoma and the rare pleural (and peritoneal) mesothelioma – is certain. What is not clear, however, is how much exposure is needed – and to what type of asbestos – before either of these cancers are liable to be produced. The use of asbestos has rocketed since the end of the Second World War. Mining began in 1878, and by 1940 world production had risen to about 350,000 tons; by 1962 to nearly 2,000,000 tons, without counting that produced in the U.S.S.R. It is now used in many articles of everyday life – in ceilings, walls and floors and in the brake-shoes and clutch linings of cars. According to Hendry (1965) it has 1,000 separate uses.

Unfortunately small particles flake off, find their way into the inspired air, and are eventually deposited in the lungs. Until recently the discovery of asbestos bodies at autopsy was a rare event; now, by more intensive search, and presumably also because of their greater prevalence, asbestos bodies have been seen in the lungs of half of all men over fifty years of age coming to autopsy in hospital (Gilson, 1966). If then small amounts of asbestos are capable of causing cancer, the asbestos risk can no longer be regarded as a specific occupational hazard of a few men employed in mining or in the asbestos textile factories, but it will have become a risk (albeit a small one) for town dwellers throughout the world.

The general question of whether a threshold exists below which no dose of a carcinogen produces a cancer is discussed in chapter 5. Here I shall consider only the data that refer specifically to asbestos. So far as bronchial carcinoma is concerned, there are several reasons for thinking that it requires both prolonged and heavy exposure. It has been reported characteristically in association with asbestosis – particularly by the Chief Inspectors of Factories (Ministry of Labour, 1965) who have recorded 169 cases in 40 years – lung cancer being present in 33 per cent of autopsies on men with asbestosis and in 14 per cent of similar autopsies on women. Knox, Doll, and Hill, who studied the changes brought about in an asbestos textile factory by the introduction of the Asbestos Regulations in 1931, found that when the risk of lung cancer was high, all cases occurred against a background of asbestosis. When asbestosis had practically disappeared, the association was lost and the incidence of lung cancer was approximately normal. In contrast to these findings, Selikoff and his colleagues in the United States observed an increased death rate from lung cancer among men working with asbestos in the building industry, without there having been any evidence of clinical asbestosis. Asbestosis, however, is not an 'all-or-none' condition. The definition is empirical, and the present evidence really means little more than that a recognizable risk occurs only when the exposure to asbestos is intense. In all these series, the vast majority of cases have been described as ordinary bronchial carcinomas. This condition is so common that the recognition of a small extra risk is extremely difficult and requires the study of many thousands of men for many years. It is natural, there-fore, that bronchial carcinoma due to asbestos should appear to be linked with the presence of asbestosis.

The position with regard to mesotheliomas of the pleura is different. This condition is normally so rare that even a small absolute risk can be rapidly detected once it has been envisaged. Altogether 302 asbestos mesotheliomas have now been described, the great majority in South Africa and the United Kingdom (Gilson, 1966). Not all have occurred in asbestos workers, but residence near a mine or close to a factory, or even in the same house as an asbestos worker, appear to have been sufficient to produce the disease – and asbestosis has seldom been present. But why hasn't the disease been found more often among men who were heavily exposed? The answer is not clear. Some cases may have occurred and not been recognized; but the more important reason would appear to be the long induction period of approximately forty years that characterizes the condition. Few of those who were heavily exposed can have survived long enough to develop it.

Mesothelioma can, it appears, develop after exposure to white asbestos (chrysotile) alone; but large numbers of cases have been described only in relation to blue asbestos (crocidolite). This is particularly obvious in South Africa, where 110 of 120 cases can be traced to the crocidolite area of north-west Cape Province, none being related to the amosite (or brown asbestos) mines of the Transvaal and none to the chrysotile mines in Swaziland (Wagner, 1965). Whether bronchial carcinoma is also produced more easily by crocidolite remains to be shown. The difficulty in this case is that the risk has been demonstrated in relation to the use of asbestos and not to its mining, and asbestos workers have seldom been exposed to one type of asbestos alone. It is clear, however, from British experience, that a high risk can occur when the asbestos used has been almost wholly chrysotile.

Other specific occupational risks of lung cancer have little general relevance (apart from those due to *ionizing radiations* and *ultraviolet light* which have been referred to previously, p. 54 and p. 58). Risks have been demonstrated in the *refining of nickel*, and *manufacture of chromates*, exposure to *inorganic arsenic compounds*, and the *manufacture of mustard gas*. Smaller risks may also be associated with some (unspecified) types of *metal mining* in the United States, with *haematite mining* in England, and with *gold mining* in Rhodesia.

Some of these risks, notably those arising from the refining of nickel and the manufacture of chromates, have been considerable. Twenty to 25 per cent of the employees involved have died of lung cancer, and this at a time when lung cancer was a relatively rare disease in the country as a whole. The risks were, however, confined to the men who treated the primary ore and carried out the early stages of the refining process, and there is no reason to suppose that contact with either pure nickel or soluble chromates carried any risk in ordinary life.

For many years lung cancer developing in men who worked on the carbonyl process of nickel refining was the only type of industrial lung cancer to be prescribed as an industrial disease. It is ironical that it should now appear that the carbonyl process itself was probably completely safe. The situation, however, has its tragic side, for the preliminary parts of the refining process were gradually transferred to Sudbury, Ontario, where the ore originated, and they took with them the specific occupational hazard, while the precautions against the disease were concentrated on Wales.

Of the other agents, arsenic is one of the most likely to have any general relevance. It exists as an impurity in many substances used in everyday life, and arsenicals have been used widely as pesticides. Its presence in coal leads to its regular addition to the atmosphere, where it may reach a concentration of 0·1 µg As_2O_3 per cubic metre. Its use as an insecticide on tobacco leaves resulted in its presence in cigarettes, and until the early 1950's when it largely ceased to be used an average of 0·15 mg As_2O_3 was volatilized with every packet of twenty ordinary British cigarettes. Satterlee and Buechley have, indeed, attributed the carcinogenic effect of atmospheric pollution and of cigarette smoke to their content of arsenic; but the figures are against them. Even immense quantities of arsenic in the air of the order of 1,000 µg per cubic metre, such as were inspired by the workers in a small sheep dip factory in Berkhamsted, gave rise to only a small number of cases of lung cancer (Hill and Faning, 1948). Many of these workers showed gross signs of arsenicism and it seems unlikely that any recognizable effect would be produced with lower doses insufficient to give rise to clinical signs in the skin. Other workers who have developed lung cancer as a result of exposure to arsenic include the vineyard workers of the Moselle, many of whom showed clinical arsenicism; and arsenic, in conjunction with nickel and other metals, may have been partly responsible for the hazards of nickel refining in Wales and of cobalt smelting in East Germany.

All these agents – atmospheric pollution, gasworks' fumes, atmospheric radon, asbestos, nickel and chrome ores, arsenic and mustard gas – must be presumed to reach the bronchial mucosa via the inspired air (except perhaps arsenic, some of which may be concentrated in the bronchial mucosa after absorption from the gut). All of them must, therefore, pass through the nose or mouth, the oropharynx, the larynx and the trachea, and it might be thought that they would produce cancers of these organs as well. In fact, only a few of them do so, and these highly selectively. The most striking association is between bronchial carcinoma and carcinoma of the maxillary antrum and ethmoid sinuses in nickel workers. Antral, and especially ethmoid, cancer are rare diseases, and the observation that 8 per cent of deaths among nickel workers was at one time due to these two cancers indicated without question the existence of a specific cancer hazard. None of the other agents have produced cancer of the nasal sinuses, not even the agent responsible for chromate cancer, despite the fact that benign ulcers of the nasal septum are common among chromate workers. Only one other occupation is known to have produced nasal cancer, namely the *manufacture of isopropylene**. In this case, there has not apparently been any concomitant risk of bronchial cancer, but the nasal cancer risk was recognized early and changes were made in the manufacturing process, so that the bronchial cancer risk may have been eliminated before it was recognized. The only other cancers attributable to these inspired carcinogens are a few cases of cancer of the larynx among the mustard gas workers in Japan, the meso-theliomas of the pleura and peritoneum in men and women exposed to asbestos, and cancer of the skin in the arsenic workers of Berkhamsted and in the vineyards of the Moselle.

The recognition of the special occupational hazards of cancer of the skin and scrotum was the foundation stone on which modern knowledge of chemical carcinogenesis was built. The observations of Pott on cancer of the scrotum in *chimney sweeps*, of Volkmann on cancer of the scrotum and skin in *tar workers*, and of Wilson on cancer of the scrotum in *cotton spinners* exposed to shale oil, led directly to the synthesis of the first known pure carcinogen, and to the isolation of 3:4-benzpyrene from tar, the first carcinogenic chemical to be obtained from a natural product. These observations form part of the history of medicine and there

* A recent report suggests that there may also have been a risk among furniture makers in Buckinghamshire (Acheson, Hadfield, and Macbeth, 1967).

is no need to emphasize them here, save to note that the experimental observations took the human findings as their starting point. At this time, and with all that is now known about carcinogens in the products of coal combustion, it would seem absurd to question the causal significance of the original observations on chimney sweeps. Yet they were questioned – and not wholly without justification – for many years. No one could repeat them on the Continent, and it seemed as reasonable to regard the cancers as being due to some feature of English life as to the soot itself. One ingenious explanation, which appealed to Hirsch, was that British sweeps sold the soot; to separate the soot from chimney rubble it had to be sieved, and it was suggested that the resulting friction rubbed the grime into the scrotum.

Not all occupational hazards have yet been recognized and some cancers of the scrotum or of the exposed skin continue to occur which cannot easily be attributed to tar or allied substances or, in the case of cancer of the exposed skin, to sunlight. A disproportionate number occur among engineering workers, and many of these can probably be attributed to the lubricating oils which have been used in the industry and which have contained substances carcinogenic to the skin of mice.

An important series of observations, the implications of which have not yet been fully realized, concerns the incidence of cancer of the bladder among men exposed to α- and β-naphthylamine, benzidine and xenylamine. As with cancers of the skin and scrotum in tar workers, observations of the effect in man led to laboratory investigation, and the carcinogenic effect of a whole class of aromatic amines was discovered when Hueper and his colleagues induced bladder tumours in dogs by the oral administration of commercial β-naphthylamine. Eventually it was realized that previous attempts to produce tumours experimentally had failed because different animals metabolized the substances in different ways, and that the carcinogenic effect was produced by a metabolite of the original substance and not by the substance itself.

The survey undertaken by Case and his colleagues on behalf of the Association of British Chemical Manufacturers, showed that the risk was highest among men exposed to β-naphthylamine, among whom it was estimated that over 50 per cent would eventually develop the disease; but it was also substantial among men exposed only to α-naphthylamine or benzidine. In the small group of fifteen men who had been employed as distillers of β-naphthylamine, all developed the disease, indicating that all are susceptible if they are exposed to a sufficient dose.

These chemicals were made largely for use as intermediaries in the *manufacture of dyestuffs* and were made harmless in the process. Some, however, were purified and sold as fine chemicals for laboratory use, and some were made into compounds for use in other industries. The manufacture of β-naphthylamine was stopped as soon as the danger from it was appreciated, but the other chemicals continued to be made until recently, albeit under strictly controlled conditions, and the pure chemicals, or compounds containing them, continued to be imported. The question arises, therefore, how far the risk may have spread outside the chemical industry. According to Case, textile printers have used α-naphthylamine and benzidine for developing dyes on cloth; benzidine has been used in medical practice as a test for the presence of blood; α-naphthylamine has been used as a reagent in testing water supplies and the effluents of some electroplating processes; and rat-catchers have been exposed to α-naphthylamine, present as an impurity in the rat poison, alpha-naphthyl-thio-urea (Antu). No surveys have, however, been made of any of these exposed groups which would reveal whether they had suffered a specific risk.

The most important groups to have been exposed are *rubber workers* and *men in the cable industry*, who have used large quantities of rubber until recently when plastics were substituted for it. Exposure arose from the fact that antioxidants, which were put into rubber to stop it perishing, were sometimes made from α- and β-naphthylamines and contained some of these substances as impurities. The extensive use of these compounds was stopped when the chemical risk was appreciated, but small amounts continued to be used. The modal induction period for these tumours is fifteen to twenty years, and it is not surprising that new cases should have continued to occur. Some diminution in the risk would, however, have been expected, and it is disturbing that Case should report that the excess mortality among rubber workers has remained at about the same level for the last thirty years. It may be, therefore, that the risk in these workers is principally due to some other, and hitherto unsuspected, class of carcinogenic chemicals.

A small risk of bladder cancer apparently also occurs among *gasworkers*. It has long been known that β-naphthylamine is present in both coal tar and gas-works pitch, and Battye has now shown that small amounts, equivalent to about 0·2 γ per 100 cu.m., can be recovered from retort house air. The amount present is minute and yet it appears to be sufficient to double the mortality from bladder cancer in the retort-house workers.

Whether *benzene* can produce leukaemia is less clear. Animal experiments have been negative, and the evidence consists entirely of case histories, many of which are, however, extremely striking. Benzene has been used widely, and variably, in many different occupations both in small factories and by individual workers, and it would be extremely difficult to define a population at risk and to follow it up for any length of time. More than sixty cases of leukaemia have been described in benzene workers, many of which have occurred following episodes of marrow aplasia. The most impressive evidence, however, is the frequency with which the leukaemias have been described as 'erythroleukaemia'. This rare cytological type does not normally represent more than one or two per cent of cases in any clinical series and the fact that twenty per cent of the cases in benzene workers are classified in this way strongly suggests the existence of some special aetiological relationship.

So far, I have considered only urban residence and occupation as the cause of local or group hazards. Many other causes are possible, but the evidence to implicate them varies from incomplete to rudimentary. The most interesting evidence relates to Burkitt's lymphoma. Pathologists still argue whether this tumour should be regarded as a specific disease entity; but the question was settled, so far as epidemiologists were concerned, when Denis Wright showed that he could pick out cases with the characteristic clinical features solely by examining sections from a mixed group of childhood lymphomas and reticulosarcomas.

The disease occurs commonly only in Africa and in New Guinea and then only in areas where the temperature never falls below 16°C and the rainfall is at least 50 cm a year. This distribution closely overlaps the distribution of some virus diseases, such as 'o'nyong-nyong' in East Africa, and Burkitt and Davies therefore suggested that the tumour might be due to a virus, spread by an insect vector. Since then much other evidence has tended to support this view. Burkitt and Wright have shown that the age distribution in persons born in endemic areas is sharply peaked, with a maximum at about seven years of age, whereas in immigrants from lymphoma-free areas the age distribution is entirely different and cases frequently occur in adult life. Pike, Williams, and Wright have now shown that within one district of Uganda, selected for study because the few physicians in it have long been interested in the disease, cases are not distributed at random, but that they spread year by year from one part to another and back to the original area several years later. This behaviour accords with the idea that infection occurs only when a high proportion of the population is susceptible and that the outcome of infection is the development of a tumour in only a small minority of cases.

The one piece of contrary evidence is that cases have been recognized – albeit very rarely – in children in South Africa, the United States, and Britain who have never visited these tropical areas. There is, however, nothing intrinsically impossible in the tumour being induced by a virus in one area and by another agent somewhere else. Indeed, if the tumour has more than one cause, this would serve only to bring it in line with the majority of other cancers.

The suggestion that the occurrence of cancer may be related to the *character of the soil* or of the *water supply* has been made frequently, but the evidence to support it is extremely weak. In Britain, gastric cancer tends to be commoner in areas where the water is soft, and it may be relevant that patients with gastric cancer show unusually little evidence of calcification in the abdominal aorta.

More impressive but equally incomprehensible observations have been made by Stocks and his colleagues on garden soils. Stocks took samples of soil from the gardens of houses in which deaths had occurred from any one of eight different types of cancer, and compared them with similar samples obtained by selecting addresses of houses in which persons had died from causes other than cancer, matching as nearly as possible the sex, age, and district of residence of the dead subjects in the two series. More than 750 soils were examined from twelve districts in North Wales, Cheshire, and Devonshire. In each district the average zinc content of the soil was found to be greater when death had been due to gastric cancer and the subject had lived in the house for more than fifteen years. Less consistent differences were found in relation to the chromium content of the soil, and no differences were found for the other six elements examined (cobalt, titanium, vanadium, nickel, lead and iron). When the copper content was measured subsequently the biggest differences were found in the ratio of zinc to copper.

These observations are particularly striking because they

are specific for one type of cancer and the differences appear only when the houses were inhabited by the subject for more than ten years. No hypothesis has been formulated to explain them; but stocks has pointed out that zinc and copper are biological antagonists, and that the addition of copper acetate to the diet has a strong retarding effect on the development of at least one type of experimental tumour – the hepatic tumour produced by giving p-dimethylamino-azobenzene to rats.

Personal behaviour

Cancer of the mouth is not a common type of cancer in Europe, but it is so common in some parts of Asia that it probably accounts for more than half of all cancers. Wherever it is common the habit of *chewing various mixtures of tobacco, betel and lime* is also widespread, and it needs little imagination to link the two. Until recently, however, hard facts were few. Now, thanks in particular to the work of Sanghvi, Raso, and Khanolkar in India and of Hirayama, who undertook an extensive survey on behalf of the World Health Organization, the position is changed.

Throughout a large area extending from Central Asia across India to Thailand, Malaya, and New Guinea, the percentage of persons who chew has been found to be uniformly higher in those who have developed oral cancer than in those who have not – and this is so, regardless of sex, socio-economic class, ethnic group, or country. The proportions of chewers varies according to the part of the mouth affected and is greatest for cancers of the buccal mucosa, followed closely by cancers of the lip and the anterior part of the tongue. Moreover, within the mouth there is a close anatomical relationship between the site at which the cancer develops and the place where the quid is habitually kept. This varies from country to country and from person to person – from the cheek, to behind the lip or under the tongue, and from the left side to the right. Retrospective studies of patients with oral cancer and of unaffected controls allow estimates to be made of the relative risks associated with different amounts of chewing. In every study the risk has been found to increase with an increase in the number of quids chewed per day, and it rises to a maximum in those who retain the quid in their mouth during sleep. In Hirayama's experience, the risk in this group is sixty times greater than in those who do do not chew at all.

Many difficulties, however, persist and the exact nature of the carcinogenic agent has still to be determined. There can be no doubt that the incidence of oral cancer would be reduced enormously if tobacco and betel chewing were discontinued. But what is not clear is whether it could also be eliminated by changing the nature of the quid, or by alleviating some associated characteristic such as a nutritional deficiency or the degree of dental sepsis. The frequent occurrence of buccal cancer in New Guinea, where betel-nut and lime are chewed without tobacco implies that tobacco is not essential; but the disease is also common in places where betel is omitted and the mixture is limited to tobacco and lime (for example, in Bihar). Mixtures of tobacco and lime are, however, also used widely in Afghanistan, and there the disease is apparently rare. The carcinogenic effect may, therefore, depend on the presence of some other factor, which Kmet suggests may be related to climatic conditions, and possibly to the bacterial flora in the mouth.

When *tobacco is smoked* instead of being chewed, cancer may be produced anywhere in the upper respiratory or digestive tracts or in the bladder – the risk of the different types of cancer varying with the way the tobacco is smoked. Most studies, however, have been concentrated on cancer of the lung, because of its numerical predominance and the rapidity with which the death rate attributed to it has increased. At first, comparisons were made between the smoking habits of patients with and without the disease and, although the method of inquiry varied greatly and was sometimes open to serious criticism, the results of twenty-nine studies reported from nine countries all led to broadly similar conclusions. Later, evidence was obtained from direct observation of mortality rates in groups of people whose smoking habits had been previously determined. Seven such studies have been carried out in Britain, Canada, and the United States, and the results of all of these are in close agreement with one another and with those of the previous retrospective studies on patients.

In every study the mortality from lung cancer has been higher in smokers than in non-smokers, and – where the comparisons were made – in cigarette smokers than in pipe smokers, in heavy cigarette smokers than in light, and in cigarette smokers who have continued to smoke than in those who have stopped. In cigar smokers the mortality has been only very slightly higher than in non-smokers. A close quantitative relationship has also been observed between dose and response, the mortality rate increasing with the amount smoked, from under ten to over forty cigarettes a day, and decreasing (relative to the rate in continuing smokers) with the passage of time after smoking has been stopped.

The simplest interpretation of these findings is that cigarette smoking is a cause of the disease; and this interpretation has been accepted by all the scientific committees that have reviewed the results. It must be remembered, however, that the observations are not the result of planned experiments. The subjects have chosen their smoking habits themselves, and the possibility has to be considered that a common factor has been responsible both for the formation of the habits and for the development of the disease. A few statisticians and at least one psychologist – but not, to my knowledge any oncologists or chest physicians – believe that genetic factors may be responsible. This hypothesis is difficult to fit with the fact that the incidence of the disease fails to increase with age when smoking has been stopped, and with the rarity of the disease in non-smoking populations like the Seventh Day Adventists. Moreover, it fails to account for the great increase in mortality that has occurred in the last forty years. It can, however, be put to a crucial test by observing what happens to the mortality figures in a group of people when many of them stop smoking. If those who stop do so because they lack a genetic factor which causes both a strong desire to smoke and a predisposition to the disease, the fact that they stop will serve only to concentrate the incidence in those who continue, and will do nothing to alter the incidence in the whole group of people who were smoking originally. If, however, smoking causes the disease, the fact that some people stop will reduce the incidence in the whole group.

Such a group is, in fact, provided by British doctors whose smoking habits and mortality rates have been observed by Sir Austin Bradford Hill and myself over the last fifteen years. Preliminary results, which are summarized in Table 3, suggest that the second possibility is what has actually happened. National habits have changed very little and the national death rate from lung cancer has increased by 25 per cent, due to the increase in mortality among old people in whom cohort effects are still operating; in contrast, many doctors have stopped smoking and the death rate among doctors as a group has fallen by 30 per cent over the same period.

TABLE 3

Trends in mortality from lung cancer;
male doctors compared with all men.
(After Doll, 1966)

Population	Death rate per 100 men aged 35 to 84 years standardized for age		
	1954–57*	1958–61*	1962–64*
All men in England and Wales	1·49	1·71	1·86
British male doctors	1·09	0·83	0·76

* The rates for doctors refer in each case to periods 2 months earlier than the rates for all men.

The evidence is similar but less complete for other types of cancer. A causal relationship appears to have been established between pipe smoking and cancer of the lip, and there is fairly strong evidence that the oral, pharyngeal, laryngeal and oesophageal cancers are all about equally related to the smoking of tobacco in all forms (cigarettes, pipes and cigars). For none of these cancers are the quantitative relationships as strong as for cigarette smoking and cancer of the lung, and for these cancers there is the added difficulty of distinguishing the effect of smoking from the equally, or more, important effect of alcohol.

For cancer of the bladder there is a weak association with cigarette smoking alone, and the possibility of a causal relationship must be seriously considered. That the relationship may be causal is supported by the fact that papillomas of the bladder have been produced experimentally by painting tobacco tar on the oral mucosa of mice, and by the fact that the incidence of the disease is tending to rise in many countries.

Whether the effect of *alcohol consumption* in producing cancer is due directly to the alcohol itself or to some other factor associated with it – including possibly a dietary deficiency – is uncertain. Alcohol has never been shown to be carcinogenic in laboratory experiments, and it is difficult to see how such a simple and easily metabolized organic substance could be a carcinogen. The epidemiological evidence is, however, strong; it is less complete than for tobacco, but even so it is difficult to interpret in any other way.

Two types of evidence have been obtained. First, the mortality from cancers of the mouth, pharynx, larynx and oesophagus has been found to be higher in groups of people who, on average, drink more. In England, the mortality has been higher in men employed in making alcoholic drinks than in other occupations. In France, the mortality in different départements correlates closely with the consumption of alcohol per head of population in that area; and in other parts of Europe, the mortality in different countries correlates with similar figures for national consumption. Secondly, retrospective studies show that a higher proportion of patients with cancers of the upper respiratory and digestive tracts give a history of heavy drinking than of control patients with other conditions. To some extent this is due to the fact that heavy drinkers tend to be heavy smokers, and this can account for the whole association between alcohol consumption and cancer of the lung. Wynder and his colleagues in the United States and Schwartz and his colleagues in France have, however, shown that it fails to account for the observations on patients with cancers of the mouth, pharynx, larynx, and oesophagus. For these conditions the incidence among men who drank heavily (defined as drinking more than six ounces of whisky or its equivalent a day) is estimated to be about ten times greater than in men who drink no alcohol at all.

In Europe, Australasia and North America, alcohol consumption is also a major factor in the production of primary carcinoma of the liver. In these countries, primary carcinoma of the liver is an extremely rare disease and when it occurs in adults it is nearly always secondary to cirrhosis. All types of cirrhosis which result in the destruction and regeneration of liver cells predispose to carcinoma and, as alcohol can lead to 'post-necrotic' cirrhosis, it is also a cause of liver carcinoma.

For some other cancers, we know how to remove the cause, even though we have no idea what the cause is.

Cancer of the penis, for example, never occurs if complete *circumcision* is performed during the first few weeks of life – irrespective of the child's genetic background or the culture in which he is subsequently educated. Performed later in life the operation is less effective. In India and East Africa the disease is common; but it is less common in Moslems who are circumcized at puberty than in Hindus, and is less common in the circumcized African tribes than in the uncircumcized. Circumcision is, however, not the only method of protection. The disease is rarely reported in some of the uncircumcized tribes (for example the Karamajo) and is uniformly rare outside the tropics. In England, the mortality from cancer of the penis is inversely related to ascending social class and it seems probable that the incidence can be closely related to the lack of facilities for physical cleanliness.

Cancer of the cervix uteri provides another example. It practically never occurs in nuns, and is presumably related to some aspect of *sexual experience*. Many studies have been designed to investigate this relationship in the last twenty years, but no prospective studies have been undertaken and the reports have generally been limited to a comparison of histories given by cancer patients with those given by selected groups of control patients with other disorders. Since the inquiries have been concerned with intimate details of the patients' sexual experience, the control patients have often been selected from women attending gynaecological clinics, and it is doubtful whether the information has been adequately representative of the population from which the cancer patients were drawn. Despite this defect, a few salient facts have begun to emerge. First, the disease is commoner in married women than in single, and in single women who have had sexual intercourse than in those who have not. Secondly, the risk of the disease is greater the younger the age at marriage or at first intercourse. Thirdly, the risk is greater in women who have had two or more marriages, or are widowed or divorced, than in women whose first marriage is unbroken. Fourthly, the risk appears to increase with an increase in parity; multiparity is, however, closely associated with age at marriage and when age at marriage is taken into account the association with parity disappears. Fifthly, the risk increases with descending social class, the disease being commonest in the poorest sections of the community.

The association with multiparity was observed many years ago, and it used to be thought that the disease was due to trauma in childbirth and that it could be prevented by good obstetric care. This, however, is clearly untrue, and it appears that the disease is related to some more immediate aspect of sexual intercourse. What this aspect is remains unknown. An obvious possibility is that the disease is related to intercourse with an uncircumcized male, and that the risk is increased by lack of physical cleanliness. The disease is rare in Jewesses, irrespective of where they live or their country of origin*. It is also less common in Moslem women than in Hindus or Christian women indigenous to the same country, and less common in Fijians than in Indians living in Fiji. In all these examples

---

* The most recent evidence from Israel suggests that this may not be true of Jewesses of North African origin who have experienced a risk of cervical cancer comparable to that of the rural population of England and Wales (Steinitz, 1967).

the disease is less common in communities in which the men are circumcized than in corresponding communities in which they are not. Studies of women in non-Jewish communities in the United States and Britain have, however, failed to provide any consistent evidence that affected women are characteristically married to uncircumcized men, and the rôle of circumcision remains in doubt. It is notable, however, that the disease is rare in the meticulously clean Parsees, despite the fact that the men are uncircumcized, and that the incidence in England is lower than anywhere else in the world apart from Israel.

Iatrogenic Factors

A few cancers – and only a minute proportion of the total – are iatrogenic in origin. Those due to *ionizing radiations* from the use of radiotherapy or thorotrast have been referred to previously, but other cases must be added which are due to diagnostic radiography and the use of radio-active isotopes. Direct evidence of the effect of the small doses received from these sources is available only for the cancers of childhood that follow irradiation *in utero*. This evidence has been discussed in chapter 2 (p. 19), and suggests that perhaps seven per cent of all the main types of cancer in children under ten years of age have been due to this cause. Retrospective study of patients' histories provides some slight evidence that diagnostic radiography produces a very small proportion of the case of myeloid leukaemia in adults, but otherwise the conclusion depends entirely on theoretical considerations and extrapolation from the effect of doses that are several orders of magnitude larger.

Arsenic, which has been mentioned as an occupational factor, has certainly also caused cancer when given medicinally. The classical examples could hardly be contested as the cancers occurred on the palm of the hand – an otherwise almost completely cancer-free site – and were accompanied by gross signs of arsenicism. The long-continued use of inorganic arsenic by mouth was, however, also associated with cancers of other parts of the skin, particularly when used for the treatment of psoriasis, and it is possible that it also produced a few cases of bronchial carcinoma. In the latter case, the most striking evidence has been that patients with arsenicism who developed bronchial carcinoma were unusually light smokers.

Chlornaphazine (dichlor-diethyl-β-naphthylamine) has been used in the treatment of multiple myeloma and is converted to β-naphthylamine in the body. It is, therefore, not surprising that six out of twenty patients who received doses of 100 to 175 g. and five out of eight who received higher doses, should have developed tumours of the bladder.

The evidence that points to *liquid paraffin* as a cause of a small proportion of cases of cancer of the stomach, colon and rectum is weak. Boyd and I found that a higher proportion of patients with these cancers had used liquid paraffin regularly over a long period than of patients with lung cancer or other non-gastro-intestinal disease. Fluorescent substances used to be present in liquid paraffin and this presumably indicated the presence of polycyclic hydrocarbons. The finding is, however, of dubious significance as it is not possible to produce gastro-intestinal cancer experimentally by giving this type of carcinogen by mouth. Polycyclic hydrocarbons, however, readily produce cancer of the skin and there is ample evidence that exposure to them in tar and other combustion products of coal give rises to occupational skin cancers in men. It is therefore, not surprising that a few cases of cancer of the skin should have appeared in such unusual sites as the thigh after the prolonged application of *ointments containing coal tar* (for example, liquor picis carbonis, BP). It is, perhaps, more surprising that the number is not larger.

Several cases of leukaemia have been described following the use of *butazolidine*, and in one series of patients with leukaemia an unusually high proportion were found to have been given butazolidine previously. The numbers were not large and confirmation needs to be sought in other series.

Many other drugs have been suspected of carcinogenic activity, including particularly the iron dextran *imferon*, *urethane*, *isoniazid*, *griseofulvin*, *oestrogens*, and *oral contraceptives* containing both oestrogens and progestogens. All have produced cancers in animals, though often only with much larger doses than are normally given to man. Human evidence has not been obtained, despite the fact that some of the drugs have been used extensively for many years and that in one case the presumed effect – a local sarcoma at the site of injection – should be easily recognizable.

Predisposing Diseases

But if medical treatment is the cause of some cancers, the lack of it is the cause of more. Many conditions that are not themselves a direct manifestation of the cancer process predispose to its development, and may be regarded as a cause of cancer in the sense that their treatment would prevent its subsequent occurrence. Such conditions include tropical ulcers of the skin, ulcerative colitis, cirrhosis of the liver, clonorchiasis and schistosomiasis.

Tropical ulcers are the immediate preceding cause of a large proportion of all squamous cell carcinomas on the legs and feet of the dark-skinned inhabitants of tropical countries, and the clinical association is so clear that it needs no statistical analysis. The ulcers originate from minor trauma and are produced by infection with the same organisms as are responsible for cancrum oris and Vincent's angina (S. schaudinni and F. fusiformis). Malnutrition may facilitate their development. They are so common in some parts of Africa that they account for possibly a third of all new hospital patients. Antibiotics have revolutionized their treatment and the use of antibiotics, coupled when necessary with excision and skin grafting, provides one of the simplest and most effective methods of preventing a common and serious type of cancer throughout a large part of the world.

Follow-up studies of patients with *ulcerative colitis* show that the incidence of cancer of the colon is some ten to twenty times greater in these patients than in the normal population. Cancers occur particularly in patients whose whole colons have been affected, when as many as 50 per cent may eventually develop the disease. They may occur many years after all colitic symptoms have subsided and it is uncertain whether medical treatment is effective in preventing the development of cancer. There is, however, no doubt about the prophylactic effect of total colectomy.

Cirrhosis of the liver has been referred to previously in relation to the carcinogenic effects of alcohol. Cancer of the liver is, however, also associated with other types of cirrhosis and, in Britain and other countries where the incidence of primary liver cancer is low, the disease practically never occurs in a histologically normal liver. It is one of the principal causes of death in patients with haemochromatosis, and commonly occurs in cirrhotic livers following infective hepatitis. In tropical countries, in which the incidence is high, liver cancer is usually associated with the post-necrotic form of cirrhosis, but an appreciable proportion of hepatomas occur in otherwise normal livers, and it seems probable that the same agent causes both cirrhosis and the cancer.

In areas where there is a high incidence of cholangiocellular carcinomas (southern China and other parts of south-east Asia) infestation of the bile ducts with the liver flukes *Clonorchis sinensis* and *Opisthorcis viverni* is common and this infestation is presumably a cause of the disease.

The relationship between *schistosomiasis* and cancer of the bladder is more controversial. Cancer of the bladder is one of the principal types of cancer in some of the countries in which schistosomiasis is common (for example, Egypt and Mozambique), and in these countries it has frequently been reported that infestation with S. haematobium is more frequent in patients with bladder cancer than in patients with other diseases. The difficulty in assessing the reports is to be sure that the intensity of investigation has been the same in the different groups of patients. The diagnosis of infestation can be made by means which vary from examination of a single urine specimen for ova to alkali digestion of the bladder at autopsy; and the proportion of subjects infested varies substantially according to the method of diagnosis adopted. Several series are, however, now available in which we can be reasonably sure that the diagnostic methods were comparable – ranging from Ferguson's original autopsy studies at the Government Medical School in Cairo in 1911 to Mustacchi and Shimkin's studies on 1,500 patients newly admitted to an American Mission Hospital in Egypt in 1958 – and these enable us to estimate that the disease is some three or four times commoner when infestation is present. The conclusion is, moreover, strengthened by the observation that the proportions of the different histological types of bladder cancer vary – the ratio of squamous to transitional types being relatively high when infestation is present.

The many other diseases associated with the development of cancer include pernicious anaemia, gastric ulcer, chronic bronchitis, and possibly, respiratory tuberculosis. Gastric cancer is three times commoner in patients with *pernicious anaemia* than in the population as a whole; but the association is presumably incidental in the sense that both diseases are caused by factors that produce atrophic gastritis. Certainly there is no evidence to suggest that the treatment of the anaemia has any effect on the subsequent risk of developing cancer. Whether *gastric ulcer* falls into the same category is less certain. The old belief that gastric cancer commonly developed in a long-standing chronic gastric ulcer is wrong. Many of the 'chronic ulcers' found in association with gastric cancer in pathological specimens must have been produced by the cancer, and not the reverse. Follow-up studies of patients with gastric ulcer agree in showing that the risk of developing malignant disease is only slightly above normal, and that many of the cancers that do occur develop in parts of the mucosa away from the ulcer. A few develop at the site of the ulcer many years later, when there is no possibility that the original diagnosis was mistaken, and it is probable that there is some small risk of malignant degeneration in a long-standing ulcer. The size of the risk is, however, insufficient to warrant prophylactic gastrectomy on a wide scale, if it is not needed for other reasons.

Many cases of lung cancer develop against a background of *chronic bronchitis*, and several studies have shown that people with a chronic cough are somewhat more likely to develop bronchial carcinoma than people without. These results are difficult to interpret, because cigarette smoking is a common cause of both diseases and, for this reason alone, an association would be bound to occur. Attempts have been made to standardize for smoking habits; but this is not easy to achieve and, as has been mentioned earlier, it is certainly not enough simply to compare groups of people who fall into the same broad categories of light, moderate, or heavy smokers. Chronic bronchitis may predispose to cancer, or it may delineate a group of people whose bronchi have been subjected to an unusual amount of cigarette smoke. In either case, the absence of chronic cough is no safeguard; and in really heavy cigarette smokers the risk of cancer is about the same, irrespective of whether they have a long-standing cough or not.

Several investigations have suggested that *respiratory tuberculosis* – or the scars left by healed tuberculosis – may also be a factor in the development of lung cancer. Pathological studies have demonstrated the appearance of micro-cancers in relation to old scars, but the frequency of the 'cancers' is so great that they cannot all be precursors of clinical cancer. Restrospective studies on patients with bronchial carcinoma and prospective studies on persons who have been diagnosed as have respiratory tuberculosis have given contradictory results, and a definite conclusion must await further evidence.

Envoi

A great deal of epidemiological evidence exists from which clues to causation may eventually be obtained. It is mostly reviewed in Clemmesen's masterly work *Statistical Studies in Malignant Neoplasms:* much of it, however, requires further analysis before conclusions that would be of practical value for cancer prevention can emerge. Thus I have omitted any reference to breast cancer and the possible rôles of infertility, inhibition of lactation, and differences in hormonal status, as we shall have much more precise information about them when current studies are finished. I have omitted consideration of socio-economic class in relation to gastric cancer, because the implications of this factor are so wide that it is difficult to know what aspect is relevant to the production of the disease; and I have made no reference to trauma, which may well be a factor in the production of melanomas, because the evidence is so confused. There is, in fact, hardly any type of cancer for which some epidemiological evidence could not be cited and, however shaky it may be in individual cases, the sum of the evidence points firmly to the conclusion that cancer as a whole is largely preventible.

In this review, I have confined myself to evidence that directly concerns the development of cancer in man, and have in consequence made no reference to the exciting possibilities that have been suggested by laboratory research. In recent years many substances that occur naturally in plants, or as a by-product of fungal infestation, have been shown to be carcinogenic in animals, and epidemiologists have been presented with the opportunity of seeing whether the distribution of these substances can be related to the distribution of any particular type of cancer in man and, more specifically, whether affected individuals can be shown to have had any unusual exposure to them. Such substances include aflatoxin and other metabolites formed by fungi on food stored under hot and humid conditions, pyrrolizidine alkaloids in species of Senecio, Crotaloria and Heliotropium plants, oestrogens in some clovers (for example, miroestrol in Pueravia mirifica), and an unidentified substance in bracken which causes cancer of the intestine.

Other substances, which are not carcinogenic in themselves, liberate carcinogens on passing through the body – cycasin, for example, liberating the powerful carcinogen methylazoxymethanol when broken down by bacteria in the gut. The list is already long and it will surely be rapidly lengthened. That one or other of the substances on it should be related to the occurrence of some of those human cancers which, like cancer of the oesophagus, cancer of the liver, and Kaposi's sarcoma, occur with high frequency in geographically limited areas, would seem a reasonable expectation.

Chapter 5

THE DOSE-RESPONSE RELATIONSHIP

Anyone concerned with the prevention of cancer has to face three problems of paramount importance. First, he must decide whether laboratory evidence of carcinogenicity in animals is to be taken as indicating a similar effect in man. This is probably the most difficult problem of all, as the only rule we can be certain of is that different species may react differently. The man who allows a substance that produces cancer in mice to be introduced into human food as a preservative carries a heavy load of responsibility if it should subsequently prove that the substance also produces cancer in man; but the load may be even heavier if, by rigid adherence to rules, he prevents the testing of a new drug that could relieve suffering on a large scale. That problems of this sort present a real dilemma is illustrated by the fact that African children are today suffering from malnutrition which could have been relieved by promoting the sale of ground nut meal, and that plans for doing this were abandoned for fear that small amounts of aflatoxin in it might cause cancer of the liver. In the absence of epidemiological evidence, a decision must be taken on the basis of theoretical knowledge; and, vital though it is, the problem of how to take this decision is outside the scope of this book.

The second problem lies in the interpretation of the results of observations on man, and in the decision as to whether an observed association is spurious or real, incidental or causal. It is, of course, always possible to take the standpoint of the Oriental historian who was

93

asked at a recent international conference what he thought was the most important result of the French Revolution and replied that it was too early yet to say; but this is no help to the Medical Officer of Health and, in practice, it is not usually difficult to reach a reasonable conclusion by the methods discussed in Chapter 2.

The third problem arises immediately the second is solved, as we then have to define the conditions under which the effect is produced. If the carcinogen produces an effect only in large doses above a certain threshold, prevention may be relatively easy. It becomes much more difficult, however, if the effect is produced down to the very lowest levels, when complete protection demands complete elimination of the factor from the environment. Let me acknowledge straight away that there can be no certain solution to this problem until we have an exact knowledge of the mechanisms by which cancer is produced. Until then we must make do with incomplete theory, analogies drawn from the results of animal experiments, and examination of the few dose-response relationships that have been observed in man.

Theoretical knowledge, in fact, tells us very little. If, as has been supposed, cancer induction were the result of a specific mutation in the genome of a somatic cell comparable in character to a mutation in a germ cell, there would be fairly strong reasons for believing that the effect of some carcinogenic agents – for example, ionizing radiations – would be proportional to dose, except, perhaps, at the lowest levels, when some degree of recovery might be anticipated. But even if this mechanism were accepted, not all agents would necessarily operate in the same way, and it might well be that some chemical or viral agents would be able to reach the relevant DNA only after they had achieved an adequate local concentration. In fact, it is clear from quantitative considerations that a point mutation in the genome of a single cell cannot comprise the whole process of cancer induction (Brues, 1960) even though point mutations may be an integral part of the mechanism in some instances.

Laboratory experiments do not get us much nearer the answer either, mainly because they are not carried out on large enough groups of animals to give any indication of the relationship at dose levels that produce cancer in less than 10 per cent of the experimental animals – the levels at which practically all human cancers occur – but partly also because of differences in the way the effect is usually measured. When animals are exposed to a carcinogen on a single occasion it is often reasonable to assess the effect of the agent by measuring the total proportion of animals affected. This effect will have different algebraic relation-ships to the dose when the proportion of affected animals is small and when it is large; when the proportion is small a linear relationship between dose and the incidence over a short period when tumours are being produced will be reflected in a linear relationship between dose and the total proportion of animals that develop the disease; when the proportion is high a similar relationship between dose and incidence will result in a curvilinear relationship with the total proportion affected, because, with the passage of time, the increased incidence rates will come to operate on populations of animals that are seriously reduced in number by the withdrawal of affected animals. To add to the difficulty different workers have used 'incidence' in different senses, laboratory workers tending to use it to imply the total proportion of affected animals, while epidemiologists use it to mean a rate of occurrence operating over a limited period of time. Here, it is used only in the latter sense, and the total proportion of affected animals is referred to as a proportion. In practice, there will be no important difference between the results obtained with the two measures of effect when the proportion affected is less than 10 per cent, but a distinct difference will appear when the proportion increases substantially above 20 per cent.

An even greater difficulty is introduced when exposure to the carcinogen is continued over a prolonged period, and particularly when it is continued throughout life. In these circumstances, tumours usually continue to appear until the end of the period of observation and the incidence is likely to continue to rise. The total proportion affected will, therefore, be dependent upon the life span of the individual subjects and anything which shortens the span – including the production of tumours – will grossly affect the proportion that is finally recorded. In these circumstances the measure of effect should always be an incidence rate at a specified time after exposure or – if it is necessary to combine all the observations into a single figure as in laboratory experiments on small numbers of animals – an index summarizing all the incidence rates. For this purpose a convenient index is the total incidence standardized for time after exposure. Unfortunately analyses have seldom been made in this way and very few of the experiments published so far can be used to provide a mathematical measure of the relationship between dose and effect.

Despite these considerations many experiments show quite clearly that the relationship is not by any means always linear. In these experiments the proportion of affected animals increases explosively with increasing dose, so that while one dose has little or no effect, a dose two or three times larger increases the proportion affected ten or twenty fold. In these circumstances the appearance of cancer may be associated with gross tissue damage and may depend on influences arising from distant parts of the body, as in the case of ovarian tumours following local irradiation and due to secondary stimulation of the pituitary. With very large doses the effect may be to reduce the incidence of tumours, and even to stop their appearance altogether, as with tumours of the thyroid in rats following doses of more than 10μC of ^{131}I.

Different results have, however, been obtained under other conditions. Druckrey and his colleagues, for example, gave daily doses of diethylnitrosamine to rats by mouth, and obtained a formula relating the daily dose to the time for tumours to appear in 50 per cent of animals which was equivalent to a linear relationship between daily dose and incidence at a given time after the start of exposure. And Engelbreth-Holm and Iversen showed that when single doses of 9,10-dimethyl-1,2-benzanthracene were painted on the skin of mice, the proportion of animals that developed papillomas was consistent with a theory of carcinogenesis that required a linear relationship with the initial dose.

Human data are even more sparse. The proportion of people who develop leukaemia has been observed following exposure to different amounts of ionizing radiations in two different situations. Brill, Tomonaga, and Heysell examined

the findings of the Atomic Bomb Casualty Commission up
to the end of 1958 and concluded that, in both Hiroshima
and Nagasaki, the data suggested a linear relationship
between dose and effect – though, with the number of cases
available for study, other relationships could not be
excluded. And Court Brown and I reached a similar conclusion from examining patients who had been irradiated
for ankylosing spondylitis. Although our study is open to the
objection that we had to add together doses received at
different times and in different parts of the spine to estimate
a mean dose for the whole spinal marrow, the conclusions
are strengthened by the fact that both studies lead to a
similar estimate of the leukaemia risk per unit dose and
both lead to an estimate of incidence in the absence of
irradiation which is very close to that actually observed.

The only other comparable observations relate to the
mortality from lung cancer in cigarette smokers. In these
studies, the carcinogen has been applied regularly over a
period of years, and the effect is recorded as an annual
mortality rate – which, in the case of lung cancer, can be
regarded as practically equivalent to incidence. Ideally,
comparison should be made after a standard duration of
exposure, but the numbers are too small to enable this to
be done with any accuracy. There is, however, evidence
that smokers of different amounts began smoking, on
average, at approximately the same age and I have, therefore, used all the age-specific rates between the ages of 35
and 84 years, and standardized them for age by the direct
method. The results obtained in three different studies –
two in the United States and one in Britain – are shown in the
Figure. In each case the data have been limited to lifelong

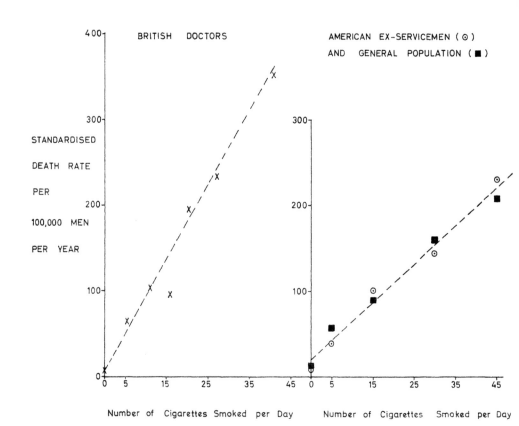

Relationship observed between lung cancer mortality and number of
cigarettes smoked per day in British and American studies.

non-smokers and to men who smoked only cigarettes and, at the time of study, were continuing to smoke. In the British study, which has been continued for thirteen years, information about smoking habits was obtained again seven years after the start of the study and the mortality in the last six years of the study was related to the information obtained from the second enquiry. In all three studies the mortality rate increased in proportion to the number of cigarettes smoked per day. It would be difficult to fit to the figures any curve that varied appreciably from a straight line, and in no case is there the slightest suggestion of a threshold dose below which no increase of risk occurs. The two large American studies reported by Hammond and by Kahn give almost identical results; but, as has been mentioned earlier, the rate of increase in mortality with increase in the amount smoked is somewhat less in the United States than in Britain.

One weakness of these data is that they fail to take account of differences in inhaling, and it seems likely from other evidence that the character of the relationship might be different if it was obtained separately for inhalers and for non-inhalers. This may be important from the point of view of carcinogenic theory, but from the practical point of view it does not affect the conclusion that people who smoke less have a proportionally smaller risk of dying of lung cancer, and that there is no evidence that any number of cigarettes per day can be regarded as 'safe'.

No other epidemiological data have been reported in sufficient detail to justify an attempt to derive a relationship between dose and effect, although there is some suggestion that a similar result might be obtained with buccal cancer and chewing habits. We may note, also the strong evidence that mesotheliomas of the pleura can be produced by minimal exposure to crocidolite asbestos (p. 64) and that childhood cancers can be produced by diagnostic irradiation in utero which cannot have exposed the foetus to doses of more than 2 to 3 rads (p. 19). In sum, the evidence points, albeit unsteadily, to the conclusion that the risk of cancer in man is proportional to the dose of the carcinogenic agent to which the individual is exposed, and that no level of exposure can be regarded as 'safe' until its safety has been proved.

Chapter 6

VARIATION IN INDIVIDUAL SUSCEPTIBILITY

In a recent symposium celebrating the centenary of Mendel's birth, Sir Gavin de Beer wrote: 'No character owes its existence to inheritance alone or to environmental factors alone. . . . No character is either innate or acquired: all are both, but in varying degrees because the degree of penetrance that genes show can be very variable.'

It would, I think, be generally accepted that this principle is as applicable to pathology as it is to normal biology, and we must enquire how far it affects the conclusions to be drawn from the facts reviewed above. In particular, we must consider the possibility that individuals who develop cancer after exposure to a particular carcinogen do so because they are susceptible to it, and that those who escape, escape because of some inherent resistance. This hypothesis, far from being of purely theoretical interest, is of concern to everyone engaged in the prevention of cancer, for it is invoked daily by people who, unwilling to involve themselves in difficult preventive measures, take refuge instead in a belief in their own personal immunity.

One possibility that has been mooted for many years is that people who develop cancer do so because they are genetically susceptible to the disease, and that exposure to a particular carcinogen serves simply to determine the site in which the cancer appears. This hypothesis, which was first stated clearly by Cramer in 1934, is held to account for the fact that the total incidence of all forms of cancer is more stable throughout the world than the incidence of cancer in any individual organ. It has the discouraging corollary that attempts to prevent cancer can succeed in postponing its onset only for a brief period, and it is still used occasionally as a justification for failing to adopt a vigorous programme of prevention.

In fact, there has long been conclusive evidence against it. First and foremost, all carefully conducted family studies agree in showing that there is no tendency for all forms of cancer, considered as an entity, to aggregate in families, and the same lack of relationship between different types of cancer has been the regular finding in all unbiased studies on twins. Secondly, there are many examples, both from industrial studies and from the study of mortality in relation to smoking, of the incidence of a particular type of cancer increasing without there being any reduction in the incidence of other types. Thirdly, the proportion of men developing cancer, who were occupationally exposed to specific cancer hazards, has been as high as 50 per cent, and in one small group described by Case (see p. 70) the proportion affected was 100 per cent. These observations, and many others, show that all people are susceptible to cancer and that cancer must be regarded as comprising a number of separate diseases characterized by the organ in which the cancer appears – a conclusion that is supported by innumerable laboratory studies on animals.

That the occurrence of cancer at particular sites is sometimes determined by heredity is certain. Family studies show that cancers can occasionally be attributed to a single gene mutation; but the number of examples in which the possession of a particular gene (or pair of genes) always leads to the development of cancer under normal environmental conditions is small, and all the genes in question are rare. In some cases, the contribution of environment is unimportant, as in some types of polyposis coli and retinoblastoma; in others, the interaction of heredity and environment is obvious, as in carcinoma of the skin developing in individuals with xeroderma pigmentosum or in Negroes with albinism.

What is of greater significance is that genetic factors sometimes affect susceptibility to the induction of common cancers, so that the incidence of a particular type of cancer varies from one genotype to another. The most noteworthy example of this phenomenon is rodent ulcer of the head and face, which is produced by exposure to sunlight; it is produced most frequently in red-haired people of fair complexion, less frequently in people of Mediterranean complexion and only extremely rarely in the Negro. Another example is melanoma of the foot, which occurs in relation to pigmented spots on the sole, the frequency of which varies greatly in different African tribes. A third example is carcinoma of the stomach, which occurs with twenty per cent greater frequency in people belonging to blood group A than in those belonging to groups O or B — and this irrespective of whether the incidence of the disease is high, as in Japan, moderate, as in Denmark, or low, as in the United States.

For most of the common cancers, however, the evidence for a genetic component is relatively weak. Even childhood cancers, which, it might be thought, are the most likely to be genetic in origin, seldom run in families. This is shown clearly by the Oxford Survey of Childhood Cancer, which covered three-quarters of the children who died of cancer in Britain under the age of 15 years in the period 1953–1960. Stewart and her colleagues obtained interviews with the mothers of over 4,000 dead children, and with the mothers of a matched control sample of living children who had not developed cancer. Among 10,000 sibs of the dead children there were 31 deaths from cancer, whereas 7 were discovered in the control series and the number expected from national mortality rates was 7·9. The excess mortality in the sibs, however, was accounted for almost wholly by cancers of the same site, as in the propositi. Eight deaths were due to leukaemia among the sibs of leukaemic children against 1·5 expected, and 16 were due to other cancers among the sibs of children who died from cancers in the same site against 2·3 expected. The corresponding numbers of discordant cancers were respectively 2 against 1·3 expected and 5 against 2·8 expected. These numbers, it must be remembered, occurred in a very large population of children, so that the excess mortality from childhood cancer that could be attributed to genetic factors was of the order of 1 in 500 (Barber and Spiers, 1964).

Twin studies provide essentially similar results. Hewitt, Lashof and Stewart obtained information about 121 twin pairs, one member of which died of cancer in an eleven-year period. Of these, 69 were like sexed and 65 of the co-twins survived birth. Only one of the co-twins developed cancer – a Wilms tumour of the left kidney – and this was similar in type and site to that from which his twin brother had suffered. The two diagnoses were, moreover, made within one month of each other. No cases of leukaemia were diagnosed in both members of a twin pair and Court

Brown and I have failed to find any examples of affected twins in the national records of leukaemia deaths in children over a period of twenty years, although thirty pairs might have been expected if concordance was complete. The failure to find any certain cases of leukaemia in both members of a twin pair in Britain is surprising as, in the United States, MacMahon and Levy found five examples in 45 twin pairs of like sex, one member of which had died of leukaemia. Perhaps the true picture is something between the two.

Stewart and her colleagues have suggested that the paucity of twin pairs with concordant cancer may be due to the genotypes which predispose to childhood cancer also carrying a high risk of embryonic or foetal death. They provide strong evidence to suggest that the number of instances in which childhood cancer occurs in one or other member of a monozygotic pair is less than expected – particularly when the pairs have not been exposed to an external carcinogenic factor *in utero*, such as ionizing radiations. But even if Stewart's hypothesis is true (and I suspect that it is), the fact remains that the occurrence of concordant tumours in monozygotic twins in childhood is the exception rather than the rule, so that even in this extreme situation non-genetic factors must be regarded as of major aetiological importance.

For adult cancers, other than the types that have been referred to previously, evidence of familial clustering is slight. The large-scale twin studies carried out in Germany by Verschuer and Kober and in Denmark by Nielsen and Clemmesen and by Hauge and Harvald showed very little excess of concordant cancers in co-twins and the excess that did occur could be accounted for almost wholly by cancers of the stomach and large bowel and those few other cancers that are known to be due to a specific allele. A few efficient family studies – and not many of the reported studies can be classed thus – have shown that gastric, breast, and lung cancer all occur in members of affected families about twice as commonly as would be expected from national figures; but whether this is due to genetic factors or to common family exposure to carcinogenic agents is uncertain. In the case of lung cancer, Tokuhata and Lilienfeld tried to answer this question by separating the smokers from the non-smokers in each family. The classification was, however, extremely crude – non-smokers including pipe smokers and ex-smokers and smokers including only current cigarette smokers – and it is unlikely to have eliminated adequately all familial differences in smoking habits. Whether heredity plays any substantial part in the production of lung cancer, other than by influencing the individual's desire to smoke, should eventually be determined by the follow-up of twins with known smoking habits, that is now being carried out in Sweden.

While, therefore, general biological principles lead us to conclude that genetic factors must play some part in determining susceptibility to the development of cancer, the human evidence weighs heavily against the belief that genetic differences in susceptibility are sufficient to account for the fact that one person develops cancer while others, who appear to be equally exposed to carcinogenic agents, do not. Thus we are left with the problem that only one man in eight who smoke 25 or more cigarettes a day dies of lung cancer, the others often living to a ripe old age. The problem is not, of course, specific to this situation, but is encountered whenever cancer can be attributed to an environmental agent. It is, however, particularly clear for lung cancer in smokers, as it can be expressed in precise quantitative terms. Part of the explanation must surely be that the attempt at quantitation is not as precise as appears at first sight. The total number of cigarettes smoked per day is not the only relevant variable; we should take account also of the age at starting to smoke, the constancy of the habit since starting, the degree of inhaling, the number of puffs taken per cigarette, and possibly also the type of tobacco, the degree of exposure to other carcinogenic agents in the ambient air, and the history of infection. Clearly this is impossible, but even if it were possible, I doubt if we should be able to specify with certainty which individual would develop the disease and which would not – still less should we be able to specify who would develop it at fifty years of age and who would develop it at seventy years. This, it may be noted, is the common experience with laboratory animals. Pure lines of genetically identical animals exposed to 'equal' doses of a carcinogenic agent never all develop cancer at exactly the same age; some develop it early, some late, and some may never develop it at all.

Kissen has suggested that psychosomatic factors may modify susceptibility, and he has brought forward evidence showing that characteristics of personality differ between affected and unaffected patients. This is certainly a theoretical possibility, but it is not biologically attractive and it remains to be shown that the personality features were not either the result of the disease or related to the sort of differences in smoking habits that have been referred to previously.

A more plausible explanation is that cancer induction is partly a matter of chance. We have not only to account for the fact that one man develops the disease while his brothers, who have been similarly exposed, do not; but we also have to account for the disease appearing in one particular part of the organ and not in another. Women who develop cancer in one breast admittedly have a higher risk of developing cancer in the other than women who were previously unaffected; but the excess risk is small and certainly not of the order that might be expected if women who develop breast cancer do so because they are specifically prone to the disease. Out of millions of clones of cells, it is unusual for more than one to develop into invasive cancer and even if we prefer to think in terms of tissue rather than individual clones the position is hardly altered. There may be, and indeed often are, widespread pathological changes in a tissue in which cancer develops. Clinical experience, however, provides many examples of successful local resection, and it is impossible to doubt that the origin of invasive cancer is commonly limited to a small part of the affected organ. All the cells of a tissue have identical genomes and we cannot attribute this variability of response to differences in inherent susceptibility, nor to any other feature that is characteristic of the organism as a whole.

Surely the most likely explanation is the play of chance. Everything we have learnt about carcinogenesis in man, tells us that the tissues are regularly bathed in carcinogenic agents before cancer appears. Whether or not changes that will eventually lead to cancer are induced in a particular part of the organ must depend on innumerable factors which determine the cellular reactions. Past exposure to other agents, the stage of the mitotic cycle, the efficiency of the homoeostatic mechanism, and the spatial distribution of the extrinsic agent are a few of them. Taken together they will have the effect of creating what appears to be a random change in one of many millions of clones. No two men can possibly have had as closely similar exposures as two clones of cells in the same tissue of the same man, and if cancer can appear in two different parts of the tissue with an interval of twenty years, it is hardly surprising that two men, apparently equally exposed, develop cancer at different ages. Nor is it surprising that some of the men at equal risk will have died of other causes before the association of many 'chance' events has finally led to the production of invasive cancer in one part of the exposed organ.

Chapter 7

THE CANCER PROCESS

When, in the last chapter, I referred to pathological changes that accompany cancer, I had in mind the type of change that Auerbach and his colleagues described in the bronchi of patients who had died of bronchial carcinoma. Auerbach removed the bronchial tree at autopsy, divided it into over two hundred portions, and examined for each subject sections from fifty-five of the portions selected to represent the whole specimen. Some abnormality was found in nearly every section (99·8 per cent). The commonest was the presence of 'atypical' cells, the nuclei of which resembled the nuclei of neoplastic cells. Many sections showed a thickened epithelium with loss of cilia and, in 11 per cent of sections, lesions were found that could be classified as carcinoma-in-situ. Similar, but less frequent, lesions were seen in cigarette smokers who had died of other causes – the frequency and severity varying with the amount smoked – and a completely normal mucosa was common only in non-smokers. Ex-cigarette smokers showed less severe changes than continuing smokers and, in particular, many fewer cells with atypical nuclei. In ex-smokers some of the sections showed cells with shrunken nuclei which suggested that they were disintegrating; these cells were never found in other subjects and it is possible that they represented 'atypical' cells on the point of disappearing.

'Atypical' cells and areas of carcinoma-in-situ similar to those described by Auerbach in bronchial mucosa accompany cancer in the tissues of many other organs, including the oesophagus, stomach, breast, cervix uteri, bladder and skin, and there are good grounds for believing that they may represent early stages in the development of the disease. First, the nuclei of the 'atypical' or dysplastic cells and of individual cells in carcinoma-in-situ are morphologically identical with the nuclei of neoplastic cells, many of them, moreover, possessing the same wide range of chromosome number; secondly, there is a high risk of the development of cancer in an organ in which carcinoma-in-situ has been diagnosed; and thirdly, there is independent evidence to suggest that the production of cancer is not an all-or-none event, but a process that takes place in several stages over a more or less prolonged interval.

The classical experiments of Berenblum and of Rous provided conclusive evidence of the existence of different types of factor, some of which initiate the production of cancer while others, which have little or no effect by themselves, magnify the effect of the initiating substances. Similarly, lesions produced by the application of a carcinogen were found to regress if the application was stopped, reappearing and developing into overt carcinoma if the application was renewed. No such conclusive evidence has been obtained in man, but the induction period is commonly so long that a fully developed malignant neoplasm can hardly be present throughout. Some cancers that are due, in all probability, to a specific occupational hazard appear twenty or thirty years after exposure has ceased. The rate of progression of these cancers is not notably different from that of cancers that occur soon after the initial exposure and it is difficult to see how this can be explained unless some further step is required before the appearance of the clinical disease.

None of this proves that the pathological changes that accompany cancer are early stages in its development, and it must be remembered that such changes are not found in all tissues; carcinoma of the large bowel, for example, usually appears as a localized disease in an otherwise normal mucosa. However, if even a small proportion of cancers develop as a result of a process which is influenced by a variety of factors and which, until the final stage is reached, can be reversed — or at any rate prevented from progressing — by altering the conditions of the internal or external environment, new possibilities for prevention are opened up. And if we can devise methods of testing the concept in practice, which might enable us to prevent the disease, this is a good reason for adopting it as a working hypothesis.

The greatest part of the work in this field has been in relation to carcinoma of the cervix uteri. Cytological examinations have been made of cervical smears from several million women throughout the world, and a large number of cases of carcinoma-in-situ and of asymptomatic invasive cancer have been detected. The benefits of this type of routine examination, however, are hard to assess. The detection of invasive cancer at an early stage, before it has begun to produce symptoms, is presumably an advantage; but the degree of reduction in fatality to be expected from earlier treatment will depend not only on the extent to which diagnosis can be brought forward, but also on the proportion of cancers that are from the beginning of different grades of malignancy. In the bronchi and the stomach a large proportion of cancers are highly malignant throughout, and the disease may be disseminated before symptoms are produced by the primary tumour, In these circumstances the fatality rate might not be reduced very greatly even if all cases could be diagnosed when they were asymptomatic. This, however, is a problem for clinical oncology and need not be considered further here. What has to be considered is the value of diagnosing lesions like carcinoma-in-situ that are thought to precede invasive cancer, and which, if effectively treated, could be regarded as preventing the development of the disease.

To some people, the problem is already solved. Carcinoma-in-situ, it is argued, can be detected in cervical smears from apparently healthy and asymptomatic women; a large proportion of cases have been shown to progress into invasive cancer; and cancer can be prevented in these women by removing the cervix – or, better, the whole uterus. If, therefore, all women were to be examined at frequent intervals, all cases of cancer of the cervix could be prevented.

The vital issue here is, of course, the length of time that could safely be allowed to elapse between examinations. If carcinoma-in-situ precedes the development of cancer, and if the lesion persists in this stage for five to ten years before becoming invasive, intervals of five years between examinations would be satisfactory. If, however, carcinoma-in-situ commonly regresses and cancer commonly develops without going through a prolonged in-situ stage, examinations would be needed much more often – possibly even twice a year. To decide which of these hypotheses more nearly represents the truth we need to know much more than we do now about the natural history of carcinoma-in-situ.

The extent of our ignorance of this subject was described very clearly by George Knox, who reviewed the situation at the request of the Nuffield Provincial Hospitals Trust. He took as an example the work of Petersen in Copenhagen showing that 35 per cent of patients with untreated carcinoma-in-situ developed invasive lesions over the course of fourteen years. This has often been cited as providing an accurate picture of the natural history of the disease. Knox, however, pointed out that the cases were diagnosed by biopsy and the patients presented because they had symptoms, and he added: 'If we are strict about definitions we should not infer that the same results would necessarily apply to women selected on the basis of routine cervical smears. On the one hand the act of biopsy in the Danish cases may have cured some cancers and the true rate of invasion to be expected in women without biopsy may have been higher. On the other hand, these women presented with symptoms, and because a complete removal of suspect tissue was not achieved many of them may already have had invasive carcinoma at the time of registration. Carcinoma-in-situ, in Petersen's study, is a histological appearance within the confines of a limited amount of material from a selected group of women and this is certainly not identical with the group we have in mind when discussing a population screening project.'

To obtain a proper understanding of the natural history of carcinoma-in-situ we need to know the age-specific incidence of (i) carcinoma-in-situ and (ii) invasive carcinoma, in women who are known to have been free from both conditions previously; and we need to be able to integrate the figures over life, and compare them with known figures for the prevalence of all stages of cancer (including death from the disease) at corresponding ages. No such data have yet been obtained, and without them we can have no sure base for believing that the treatment of carcinoma-in-situ will necessarily reduce the mortality from clinical cancer. We can, of course, perform the experiment and see whether it is justified by the results. The experiment, however, needs to be on such a large scale and continued for so many years that not even the intensive screening programme in British Columbia has been able to satisfy all the requirements. Despite the immense number of examinations carried out there and the high proportion of women examined, the death rate from cervical cancer has not changed. And so long as this is the case, it remains possible that the effect of screening has been to bring about earlier treatment of those slowly progressing types of cancer that would, in any case, have been cured when they presented clinically, while the rapidly growing and fatal cancers have been unaffected.

'The situation', as Knox said, 'recalls the long period of uncertainty preceding the use of BCG in this country, and the shorter period associated with poliovaccine. Evidence for their usefulness accumulated initially as anecdotes or as deductions made from pathological and physiological responses in individuals but without the solid backing of a large-scale well-planned trial. It is difficult now to criticize those enthusiasts who pressed for wide application of these measures without more ado, because with hindsight they are seen to have been right. However, to the extent that insufficient caution engendered a polemical atmosphere, and thus hindered the completion of proper trials and consequent general acceptance, the result was delay and the cost was in lives.'

An entirely different type of evidence has been obtained from the study of lung cancer in relation to smoking – or rather from the study of the effect on mortality when smoking is stopped. All the major prospective studies show that the mortality among ex-cigarette smokers falls off in relation to the rate among men who continue to smoke, that the difference is already marked within five years of the habit being abandoned, and that the ratio of the rates becomes progressively less as the period of non-smoking increases. These results have sometimes been interpreted to mean that the risk of developing lung cancer decreases when smoking is discontinued. In fact this is not the case; what appears to happen is that the risk fails to increase as it would do if smoking was continued, and remains approximately the same for a period, until it is eventually equalled by the risk among non-smokers which is steadily rising with increasing age (Doll, 1966). These results resemble those obtained by the prolonged application of a cancer-promoting agent to the skin of mice, followed by its abrupt cessation.

It is hardly possible to regard the effect of smoking as being simply the induction of the cancer process because continued smoking beyond, say, twenty-five years had a much greater effect on the absolute incidence rate than the same amount of smoking without any previous exposure. Continued smoking must, therefore, have some effect on an intermediate stage in the development of the disease, increasing the risk of the appearance of invasive cancer the longer it is continued. When smoking is discontinued the changes that have been produced are, it appears, irreversible; but their progression towards invasive cancer no longer proceeds with the passage of time, but is regulated by the occurrence (or non-occurrence) of some further event that has the same chance of occurring in any subsequent period.

In sum, all the evidence – experimental, pathological and epidemiological – points in the same direction, and it is difficult to escape the conclusion that cancer production is characteristically a composite process and not an isolated event. If this is so, the opportunities for prevention could be enormously increased. For the possibility of recognizing those people in whom the process was already advanced would allow the effective concentration on them of preventive measures that would otherwise be diffused over the population as a whole – a population which would include many persons in no real danger of developing the disease unless there was an increase in the normal expectation of life to ninety or a hundred years.

Chapter 8

PRACTICAL STEPS TO PREVENTION

'There is less hazard,' wrote Konrad Lorenz at the end of his work *On Aggression*, 'of my meeting with disbelief than of incurring the reproach of banality when I now proceed to summarize the most important inferences from what has been said . . . by formulating simple precepts for preventive measures.' The hazard in Lorenz's case was slight, but even if the measures he proposed had been as commonplace as those I am about to suggest, he would still have been justified in pointing out that the application of knowledge gained by scientific research demanded 'no less perspicacity and meticulous application to detail than were necessary to gain it.' Indeed, it sometimes appears that the more banal the conclusions the greater the skill required to act on them.

In the case of cancer, our lack of knowledge of the intimate mechanism by which the disease is produced stands in the way of attempts to prevent it. When we know how the body normally regulates cellular proliferation and understand the nature of the molecular changes that result in the breakdown of this mechanism, it may be possible to develop a simple and effective programme for preventing the disease in all its manifestations. As things now are, we have to attack each type of cancer separately, on the basis of empirical observations of the conditions under which it occurs. These, it is evident, are many and varied, and practical prevention involves interference with many of the normal activities of life. Just when intervention is justified, how far it calls for action at government level, and the price in social disturbance we can afford to pay for the elimination of a hazard to health, are matters which require fine judgement. They are seldom the concern of the medical profession alone, for although medical scientists have the responsibility for determining the facts and quantitating the risks, the formulation of a practical policy for preventing the disease often requires the participation of society as a whole.

In the preceding chapters I have outlined the extent to which observations on man justify the belief that cancer is preventible, and have described the conditions which, we have reason to believe, are responsible for a substantial proportion of the cancers that now occur. In many cases the action required is obvious and I do not propose to list each individually. I shall instead summarize the principles that have emerged, put forward practical proposals arising out of them, and discuss in detail only some of the ways in which it may be possible to influence personal behaviour.

First, it must be acknowledged that there is no sure way of knowing whether an agent is carcinogenic to man until the test is made and man himself is exposed. This is not to say that preventive action can never be taken on other grounds, but it does mean that other reasons for action are fallible. The range of carcinogenic agents thus far recognized is so wide that it is unreasonable to suppose that all have now been discovered; and it must be assumed that in an industrial society new hazards will continue to be introduced which unfortunately may take many years to recognize. The latent period between first exposure and the appearance of cancer is normally prolonged, and the existence of a small hazard may be extremely difficult to detect, particularly if the incidence of the disease is already high because of other causes. It would, therefore, be a major advance if a system could be worked out that would enable a new hazard to be detected in the minimum time.

The problem, so far as occupational hazards are concerned, could be partly solved if industrial medical officers accepted the need to maintain a detailed follow-up of all the personnel employed on the specific processes of their industry (including men who leave the industry, but excluding for the sake of simplicity those who remain in employment for only a few years). Such follow-up studies should be part of the routine responsibilities of all industrial medical officers, particularly when new substances or new methods are being brought into the process of manufacture. For the many small industries which do not have an industrial medical service, the answer might be the institution on a national scale of a system of record linkage like that introduced on a regional scale in Oxford by Donald Acheson, with the support of the Nuffield Foundation and the Ministry of Health.

We, in Britain, with our national health service and high standard of vital statistics have an unrivalled opportunity for introducing a national record linkage system. By the use of electronic computers it is possible to bring together all medical and vital statistics data relating to the birth, marriage, hospital admissions and death of an individual, so that with sufficient data for personal identification it becomes a simple matter of routine analysis to determine the incidence and mortality of cancer or any other disease in any selected group of employees.

Such a system would also contribute in other ways to knowledge of the causes of cancer. It would reveal relationships with predisposing diseases (as, for example, cancer of the colon with ulcerative colitis) and would provide a means for monitoring the effect of new methods of treatment. No matter how carefully pharmaceutical firms screen drugs they can never quite eliminate the possibility that a drug, non-carcinogenic to experimental animals of the type, and in the number, examined, may nevertheless be carcinogenic to man; nor can the 'early warning' system of recording adverse effects that has been adopted by the Dunlop Committee be expected to indicate a small effect that occurs many years after the drug is taken, and it would certainly not be able to quantitate the effect with any accuracy. To be able to detect risks of this sort rapidly and surely would be of special value: not only would it enable some cases of cancer to be prevented, but it would also avoid the banning of valuable drugs on inadequate grounds.

The second principle is that there should be no question of waiting for proof that a particular factor causes cancer in man, before acting to remove it. The nature of the subject is such that proof in the strict sense of the word is seldom obtainable. Experiments deliberately planned to *produce* cancer in man are unacceptable, though they may occasionally be carried out unintentionally – as, for example, when isoniazid was given to a randomly selected group of subjects with the object of preventing clinical tuberculosis*. Experiments to *prevent* cancer are conceivable, but the

---

* Isoniazid is a weak carcinogen for some animals; there is no evidence that it causes an appreciable amount of cancer in man in the doses normally employed, but if it does, it will be shown to do so by this experiment.

circumstances in which they are appropriate are rare. In the absence of proof decisions have to be based on analogy or on observation of an association in man which, in the light of all the ancillary evidence, seems likely to indicate cause and effect. 'Science,' Sherrington said, 'nobly can wait for an answer; common sense pressed for time must act on acceptance', and we must normally expect preventive measures to be vindicated (if at all) by their success.

It is, therefore, particularly important that preventive measures should be introduced in such a way that their results are capable of assessment. If they are introduced uniformly and halfheartedly over a whole country it may be impossible to distinguish the effect of the measures from a change in incidence due to other causes. The best hope of discovering whether atmospheric pollution is a cause of lung cancer, and incidentally of chronic bronchitis, would have been to initiate an intensive programme for the elimination of pollution in a few randomly selected cities, while allowing the rate of progress in other cities to adjust itself in the normal way. Similarly, the most practical way of determining the value of cytological screening for the prevention of fatal cancer of the cervix uteri is to carry out an intensive campaign in some cities, while in others providing a screening service only for those who ask for it. Such a policy would not be easy to carry out, but the stakes are high and the results, whether positive or negative, would be of value. That the experiment is possible is shown by the fact that a similar scheme has already been carried out successfully in another field to test the value of the fluoridation of water.

The third principle is that no dose of a carcinogenic agent, no matter how small, can be assumed to be safe. Exceptionally, a particular agent may be shown to be carcinogenic only in high doses and in defined circumstances – as appears to be the case with alcohol, which may produce its effect indirectly by association with other factors, or secondarily by producing tissue damage. Normally, however, it must be assumed that when cancer is produced in only a small proportion of subjects, as it nearly always is under human conditions, the amount produced is proportional to the dose to which the subjects have been exposed. Policy must, therefore, aim at the most complete removal of the agent that is both practicable and compatible with other relevant considerations. It would be ridiculous to demand that atomic energy workers should have such a degree of protection against ionizing radiations that the substitution of atomic energy for the combustion energy of coal was held back and the elimination of greater risks in the coal mining industry was prevented, but this kind of argument must not be used as an excuse to do less than we can. As Mayneord pointed out in a previous Rock Carling monograph, comparative risks 'serve to illuminate starkly the absurdities of the relative emphasis placed on radiation hazards relative to others, but that is all. It is still our duty to preserve the gain and minimize the risk.'

Once an occupational risk is recognized, the precautions needed to minimize exposure are usually undertaken with commendable speed by the industries principally concerned. In this way the occupational hazards of lung cancer among employees in asbestos textile factories and of bladder cancer in the British chemical industry have been largely or completely eradicated. Adequate steps are not always taken, however, to prevent the spread of the hazard to small groups of men who may come into contact with the carcinogenic agents in other ways. When β-naphthylamine was discovered to be so dangerous that the manufacture of it in this country was discontinued, it would surely have been desirable to limit its use to purposes for which no alternative was available. Yet David Wallace has reported that one of his patients purchased in London, without restriction, a hundredweight of β-naphthylamine seventeen years after the manufacture of the material in Britain had ceased. The regulations that have been introduced recently by the Ministry of Labour to control the use of the carcinogenic aromatic amines should be effective for the purpose for which they are intended; but they apply only to establishments that come under the jurisdiction of the Factories Act. They cannot affect the laboratory use of benzidine by pathologists, or the field use of poisons containing α-naphthylamine by ratcatchers. Voluntary limitation of the use of such substances is a slow and fallible process; but while outright prohibition of their use may be impracticable, it would be possible to make their manufacture or import subject to licence, and to grant licences only when the use of the substances was both approved and controlled. The use of such substances could also be discouraged by differential taxation of materials containing them.

For the control of hazards due to asbestos, such methods alone would not be adequate since the risks associated with this material are too widespread. In this case, an integrated policy will have to await the advice of the expert committees which have been set up to review the problem by the

International Union against Cancer and the International Agency for Research on Cancer. The attack could be begun, however, by requiring import licences for crocidolite, a type of asbestos which appears to be particularly dangerous and whose use is seldom essential.

The fourth principle of cancer prevention to which I should like to refer concerns the possibility of concentrating medical attention on groups of the population who are particularly liable to develop the disease. Variation in genetic susceptibility provides one such opportunity. It is valuable, for instance, to distinguish families with polyposis coli, since affected individuals almost invariably develop cancer of the colon if the colon is not removed prophylactically; and to distinguish individuals with red hair and fair complexion, since they are prone to develop cancer of the skin when heavily exposed to ultra-violet light. On the whole, however, there is little to suggest that man has much inherent variation in susceptibility to most of the individual types of cancer, and he certainly possesses no important hereditary characteristics that make him either more or less suceptible to the whole range of cancers in all organs.

A more generally useful technique is to concentrate preventive measures on high risk groups, defined by their degree of exposure to a carcinogenic agent or by the recognition that the cancer process has already developed to a nearly malignant stage in one or other organ. Thus men who have been exposed to α- or β-naphthylamine can be kept under supervision, and the presence of carcinoma-in-situ or the earliest stages of clinical cancer detected by cytological examination of urine samples; married women, particularly those who married early in life, can have regular vaginal smears for the detection of carcinoma-in-situ of the cervix uteri; and special efforts can be made to persuade men who have smoked heavily to stop smoking cigarettes. Few single advances would contribute more to cancer prevention than the extension of exfoliative cytology to enable the presence of carcinoma-in-situ in the bronchi to be recognized by examination of the sputum – that is, if bronchial carcinoma does, indeed, go through a prolonged and reversible in-situ stage. For it would surely have more effect if a man could be told that he had, say, a one in three chance of developing lung cancer in five years than it does now when he is told that he has a one in ten chance of developing the disease in thirty years.

'The public,' Trotter said, 'looks to doctors to give them absolution not exhortation', and the advice that continued good health depends on one's personal choice of daily activities is seldom welcome. It would be so much pleasanter if health could be assured by a factory's changing its method of manufacture, by drivers maintaining the engines of their lorries in better condition, or by the prohibition of a particular type of food additive. But such measures, important though some of them are, are not as important as those we need to take ourselves. Exposure of the skin to sunlight, the chewing of various mixtures of tobacco, betel and lime, the smoking of tobacco, the consumption of alcohol, sexual intercourse, and lack of physical cleanliness are all, in one way or another, related to the development of cancer and the choice between gratification and the avoidance of risk is one which only the individual can make. To make this choice intelligently, however, the individual must know the facts, and more research and more wide-spread health education are both necessary before he can be expected to appreciate them fully. To say that we must make our own choice is not, of course, to absolve national and local governments of all responsibility. The principle of government action in the field of individual health has long been accepted; morphine is banned and alcohol is deliberately taxed at a high level. If the risk is serious, we can reasonably ask governments to help by weighting the balance in favour of reducing it.

In Britain today the only risk that is sufficiently serious to justify government intervention of this type is the risk of lung cancer – a disease which can now be expected to kill one in every twelve males born, and which is responsible for 12 per cent of all male deaths between the ages of 45 and 64 years. In the past few years health education and the measures that have been taken to limit advertising have achieved a considerable success. The trend in tobacco sales has been reversed and, according to the Ministry of Health, there were nearly one and a quarter million fewer smokers in Britain in 1966 than there would have been had the smoking habits of the population remained the same as four years before. The rate of progress, however, is slow and it is doubtful if the present methods of prevention by precept will have any substantial effect on the incidence of lung cancer during the next twenty years. Any attempt to prohibit smoking would be inefficient and socially disastrous, but there are, nevertheless, opportunities for reducing the consumption of cigarettes, without impairing the individual's freedom of behaviour. There is now ample evidence to show that the smoking of cigars is less injurious than the smoking of cigarettes not only as regards cancer production but also in connexion with other illnesses. It is uncertain whether this is due to differences in the tobacco, to differences in the chemical or physical nature of the smoke, or to the fact that cigarette smokers tend to inhale whereas cigar smokers do not; and it is possible that a change from cigarettes to cigars might not have the anticipated effect if ex-cigarette smokers continued to inhale when smoking cigars. In the present state of knowledge, however, cigarette smokers would be well advised to change to cigars, if they are unable to discontinue smoking altogether. No form of education is as effective as fiscal pressure and it is a curious anomaly that taxation should still be at a higher level on cigar tobacco than on cigarette tobacco. A policy of reducing taxation on cigars while, if the national need demands it, increasing taxation on cigarettes might be unwelcome to the housewife, but it could have an appreciable effect on the expectation of life. It is certainly practicable, for it has been adopted in Holland.

Whether advertisements play any material part in maintaining the demand for tobacco is open to debate, but it is difficult to see how they can influence the choice of brand without in some measures encouraging the desire to smoke. The fact that so much effort is expended on preventing individuals from having access to marijuana while, at the same time, exhortations to smoke cigarettes continue to appear on public hoardings may well come to be regarded as one of the more remarkable inconsistencies of our age. The least that could be done, short of the banning of widespread advertising of tobacco, is to require that advertisers should pay a tax equal to the cost of the advertisements into a fund to subsidize the cost of health education.

It is doubtful if we have enough knowledge yet to justify any form of primary prevention of cancer of the cervix uteri. The incidence of the disease should be reduced if the beginning of regular intercourse was postponed to a later age than is usual at present, and this is an additional argument in favour of raising the age at marriage in countries such as India where the disease is common and marriage is permissible at fifteen years of age. In most countries, however, social pressures are all in the other direction and the fear of incurring a relatively rare disease would be unlikely to have much effect on individual action. If circumcision of the male were established as being of real prophylactic value, a case could be made out for performing the operation more freely, but the evidence is inconclusive. Education in physical cleanliness, and a public policy of providing a bath and hot water supply in every house, are so desirable for other reasons that doubts as to their prophylactic value need not prevent their inclusion in a programme for cancer prevention. Certainly cleanliness is of value in reducing the incidence of cancer of the skin and scrotum due to occupational causes and, in all probability, this also holds for cancer of the penis.

To sum up, we now know how to avoid the occurrence of a number, still relatively small, of the various types of cancer. Setting aside the possible benefits of earlier diagnosis, we might now be able to prevent about 40 per cent of the cancer deaths that occur annually in men in Britain, and a somewhat smaller proportion — about 10 per cent — in women. In addition, there is good reason to believe that a large proportion of the remaining types is, in principle, preventible, and with continued research we may learn how to prevent them within the next two or three decades. Some small residuum of cancer, due possibly to such factors as naturally occurring body radioactivity, is likely to remain until we have complete understanding of the mechanism by which cancer is produced, and possibly even beyond. As these cancers are likely to increase in incidence with age it might be argued that all we do by preventing the development of one group of cancers is to create the conditions in which others will occur a few years later. Indeed in time the development of cancer may come to be regarded as the equivalent of the inevitable accident in Shaw's *Back to Methuselah*. That time, however, is far off. The mortality from cardiovascular disease rises so rapidly in old age that even if all cancer were now prevented the male expectation of life would be increased by only two-and-a-half years. That figure is not large; but it is an average spread over a whole population of which four-fifths die of other diseases, and the man who dies of cancer loses an average of twelve-and-a-half years expected life, the woman eleven-and-a-half years. Now that infectious diseases have been brought so effectively under control, the prevention of cancer has come to mean the prevention of one of the principal causes of death in childhood and middle age. It is, for the most part, a practicable objective within the next few decades.

EPILOGUE

To be invited to review a field in which Sir Ernest Rock Carling 'had been particularly interested' is to be given virtually a free hand. His interests and enthusiasms ranged widely over the whole of surgery and medicine and it is typical of him that, a surgeon, he should have been so interested in new developments in medicine that in 1946 he became the second Chairman of the Committee of the Institute of Social Medicine in Oxford.

The creation of this Institute and the leadership of its director, Professor John Ryle, were largely responsible for arousing my own interests in epidemiology and my purpose in preparing this monograph is epitomized in the second of the Institute's three purposes: 'to investigate the influence of social, genetic, environmental and domestic factors on the incidence of human disease and morbidity.' Much of the work I have referred to was carried out by the staff of the Institute, and it must have given Sir Ernest great pleasure that the results of their work played such a large part in the deliberations of the International Commission for Radiological Protection – of which he was also Chairman for many years.

I am deeply appreciative of the honour of having been a Rock Carling Fellow; and it is a great pleasure to be able to acknowledge my indebtedness to Sir Ernest for the help which he gave Dr. Court Brown and myself in our studies on the long-term effects of radiotherapy and to the ideas with which, in Oxford, he was so closely associated.

BIBLIOGRAPHY

Acheson, E. D. (1965). The structure, function and cost of a file of linked health data. In: *Mathematics and computer science in biology and medicine*, Medical Research Council, H.M. Stationery Office, London.

Acheson, E. D., Hadfield, E. H. and Macbeth, R. G. (1967). Carcinoma of the nasal cavity and accessory sinuses in woodworkers. *Lancet*, **1**, 311.

Auerbach, O., Stout, A. P., Hammond, E. C. and Garfinkel, L. (1961). Changes in bronchial epithelium in relation to cigarette smoking and in relation to lung cancer. *New Engl. J. Med.*, **265**, 253.

Auerbach, O., Stout, A. P., Hammond, E. C. and Garfinkel, L. (1962). (1) Changes in bronchial epithelium in relation to sex, age, residence, smoking and pneumonia: (2) bronchial epithelium in former smokers. *New Engl. J. Med.*, **267**, 111 and 119.

Barber, R. and Spiers, P. (1964). Oxford Survey of Childhood Cancers: Progress Report II. *Monthly Bull. Minist. Hlth.*, **23**, 46.

Battye, R. (1966). Bladder carcinogens occurring during the production of 'town' gas by coal carbonization. Paper read to the International Conference on Industrial Medicine, Vienna, July 1966.

Berkson, J. (1955). The statistical study of association between smoking and lung cancer. *Proc. staff Meetings Mayo Clinic*, **30**, 319.

Berkson, J. (1959). The statistical investigation of smoking and cancer of the lung. *Proc. Mayo Clin.*, **34,** 206.

Blum, H. F. (1959). *Carcinogenesis by ultraviolet light.* Princeton Univ. Press, Princeton.

Boyd, J. T. and Doll, R. (1954). Gastro-intestinal cancer and the use of liquid paraffin. *Brit. J. Cancer,* **8,** 231.

Brill, A. B., Tomonaga, M. and Heyssel, R. M. (1962). Leukaemia in man following exposure to ionizing radiation: a summary of the findings in Hiroshima and Nagasaki and a comparison with other human experience. *Ann. int. Med.,* **56,** 590.

Brues, A. (1960). Critique of mutational theories of carcinogenesis. *Acta Un. int. Cancr.,* **16,** 415.

Buck, S. F. and Brown, D. A. (1964). *Mortality from lung cancer and bronchitis in relation to smoke and sulphur dioxide concentration, population density and social index.* Research Papers No. 7, Tobacco Research Council, London.

Buechley, R. W. (1963). Epidemiologic consequences of an arsenic-lung cancer theory. *Amer. J. publ. Hlth.,* **53,** 1229.

Burkitt, D. and Davies, J. N. P. (1961). Lymphoma syndrome in Uganda and tropical Africa. *Med. Press,* **245,** 367.

Burkitt, D. and Wright, D. (1966). Geographical and tribal distribution of the African lymphoma in Uganda. *Brit. med. J.,* **1,** 569.

Burrell, R. J. W., Roach, W. A. and Shadwell, A. (1966). Esophageal cancer in the Bantu of the Transkei associated with mineral deficiency in garden plants. *J. nat. Cancer Inst.,* **36,** 201.

Case, R. A. M. (1956). Cohort analysis of cancer mortality in England and Wales, 1911–54, by site and sex. *Brit. J. prev. soc. Med.*, **10**, 172.

Case, R. A. M. (1966). Tumours of the urinary tract as an occupational disease in several countries. *Ann. roy. Coll. Surgeons Eng.*, **39**, 213.

Case, R. A. M., Hosker, M. E., McDonald, D. B. and Pearson, J. T. (1954). Tumours of the urinary bladder in workmen engaged in the manufacture and use of certain dyestuff intermediates in the British Chemical Industry. *Brit. J. industr. Med.*, **11**, 75.

Clemmesen, J. (1965). *Statistical studies in malignant neoplasms.* Munksgaard, Copenhagen.

Cornfield, J. and Haenszel, W. (1960). Some aspects of retrospective studies. *J. chron. Dis.*, **11**, 523.

Cornfield, J., Haenszel, W., Hammond, C., Lilienfeld, A. M., Shimkin, M. B. and Wynder, E. L. (1959). Smoking and lung cancer: recent evidence and a discussion of some questions. *J. nat. Cancer Inst.*, **22**, 173.

Correa, P. and Llanos, G. (1966). Morbidity and mortality from cancer in Cali. *J. nat. Cancer Inst.*, **36**, 717.

Court Brown, W. M. and Doll, R. (1957). Leukaemia and aplastic anaemia in patients irradiated for ankylosing spondylitis. *Med. Res. Counc. Spec. Rep. Ser.*, No. 295, H.M. Stationery Office, London.

Court Brown, W. M., Doll, R. and Hill, I. D. (1964). Leukaemia in Britain and Scandinavia. *Path. Microb.*, **27**, 644.

Cramer, W. (1934). The prevention of cancer. *Lancet*, **1**, 1.

De Beer, G. (1966). Genetics: the centre of science. *Proc. roy. Soc. Series B.*, **164,** 154.

Doll, R. (1966). Cancer bronchique et tabac. *Les Bronches,* **16,** 3131.

Doll, R. (1967). The geographical distribution of cancer. *To be published.*

Doll, R. and Cook, P. (1967). Summarizing indices for comparison of cancer incidence data. *Int. J. Cancer,* in press.

Doll, R. and Hill, A. B. (1950). Smoking and carcinoma of the lung. *Brit. med. J.,* **2,** 739.

Doll, R. and Hill, A. B. (1952). A study of the aetiology of carcinoma of the lung. *Brit. med. J.,* **2,** 1271.

Doll, R. and Hill, A. B. (1954). The mortality of doctors in relation to their smoking habits: a preliminary report. *Brit. med. J.,* **1,** 1451.

Doll, R. and Hill, A. B. (1964). Mortality in relation to smoking: ten years' observations of British doctors. *Brit. med. J.,* **1,** 1460.

Doll, R., Payne, P. and Waterhouse, J. (1966). *Cancer incidence in five continents.* International Union against Cancer, Springer-Verlag, Berlin.

Dorn, H. F. and Cutler, S. J. (1955). *Morbidity from cancer in the United States: Part 1. Variation in incidence by age, sex, race, marital status, and geographical region.* Public Health Monograph No. 29, U.S. Government Printing Office, Washington.

Druckrey, von H., Schildbach, A., Schmähl, D., Preussmann, R. and Ivankovic, S. (1963). Quantitative analyse der carcinogenen Wirkung von Diäthylnitrosamin. *Arzneim.-Forsch.,* **13,** 841.

Dungal, N. (1961). The special problem of stomach cancer in Iceland. *J. Amer. med. Ass.*, **178,** 789.

Engelbreth-Holm, J. and Iversen, S. (1951). On the mechanism of experimental carcinogenesis. *Acta path. microbiol. Scand.*, **29, 77.**

Ferguson, A. R. (1911). Associated bilharziasis and primary malignant disease of the urinary bladder, with observations of a series of forty cases. *J. Path. Bact.*, **16, 76.**

Gilson, J. C. (1966). Health hazards of asbestos: recent studies on its biological effects. *Trans. Soc. Occupational Med.*, **16,** 62.

Haenszel, W., Loveland, D. B. and Sirken, M. G. (1962). Lung cancer mortality as related to residence and smoking histories. *J. nat. Cancer Inst.*, **28, 947.**

Hammond, E. C. (1966). Smoking in relation to the death rates of one million men and women. In: *Epidemiological study of cancer and other chronic diseases.* National Cancer Institute Monograph No. 19, U.S. Government Printing Office, Washington, pp. 127–204.

Hauge, M. and Harvald, B. (1961). Malignant growths in twins. *Acta genet.*, **11, 372.**

Hendry, N. W. (1965). The geology, occurrences, and major uses of asbestos. *Ann. N.Y. Acad. Sci.*, **132,** 12.

Hewitt, D., Lashof, J. C. and Stewart, A. (1966). Childhood cancer in twins. *Cancer*, **19,** 157.

Higginson, J. and Oettlé, A. G. (1960). Cancer incidence in the Bantu and 'Cape Coloured' races of South Africa: report of a cancer survey in the Transvaal (1953–55). *J. nat. Cancer Inst.*, **24,** 589.

Hill, A. B. (1962). The statistician in medicine. *J. Inst. Actuaries*, **88**, 178.

Hill, A. B. (1965). The environment and disease: association or causation? *Proc. roy. Soc. Med.*, **58**, 295.

Hill, A. B. and Faning, E. L. (1948). Studies in the incidence of cancer in a factory handling inorganic compounds of arsenic: I. Mortality experience in the factory. *Brit. J. industr. Med.*, **5**, 1.

Hirayama, T. (1966). An epidemiological study of oral and pharyngeal cancer in central and south-east Asia. *Bull. Wld. Hlth. Org.*, **34**, 41.

Hirsch, A. (1883). *Handbook of geographical and historical pathology*. Vols. 1-3. Translated from the second German edition; The New Sydenham Society, London.

Hueper, W. C., Wiley, F. H. and Wolfe, H. D. (1938). Experimental production of bladder tumors in dogs by administration of beta-naphthylamine. *J. industr. Hyg.*, **20**, 46.

International Commission on Radiological Protection (1966). *The evaluation of risks from radiation*. International Commission for Radiological Protection Publication 8, Pergamon Press, Oxford.

Kahn, H. A. (1966). The Dorn study of smoking and mortality among U.S. veterans: report on eight and one half years of observation. In: *Epidemiological study of cancer and other chronic diseases*. National Cancer Institute Monograph No. 19, U.S. Government Printing Office, Washington, pp. 1-125.

Kissen, D. M. (1966). Psychosocial factors, personality and prevention in lung cancer: a report on men aged 55-64. *Med. Officer*, **116**, 135.

Knox, E. G. (1966). Cervical cytology: a scrutiny of the evidence. In: *Problems and progress in medical care.* Edited by G. McLachlan; Nuffield Provincial Hospitals Trust, Oxford University Press, London.

Knox, G. (1964). Epidemiology of childhood leukaemia in Northumberland and Durham. *Brit. J. prev. soc. Med.,* **18,** 17.

Knox, J. F., Doll, R. and Hill, I. D. (1965). Cohort analysis of changes in incidence of bronchial carcinoma in a textile asbestos factory. *Ann. N.Y. Acad. Sci.,* **132,** 526.

Lawther, P. J., Commins, B. T. and Waller, R. E. (1964). A study of the concentration of polycyclic aromatic hydrocarbons in gasworks retort houses. *Brit. J. industr. Med.,* **22,** 13.

Lilienfeld, A. M. (1959). On the methodology of investigations of aetiologic factors in chronic diseases: some comments. *J. chron. Dis.,* **10,** 41.

Lilienfeld, A. M. (1959). Emotional and other selected characteristics of cigarette smokers and non-smokers as related to epidemiological studies of lung cancer and other diseases. *J. nat. Cancer Inst.,* **22,** 259.

Lorenz, K. (1966). *On aggression.* Methuen, London.

MacMahon, B. (1962). Prenatal X-ray exposure and childhood cancer. *J. nat. Cancer Inst.,* **28,** 1173.

Maxwell, T. (1879) Epithelioma in Kashmir. *Lancet,* **1,** 152.

Mayneord, W. V. (1964). *Radiation and health.* The Nuffield Provincial Hospitals Trust, London.

Merkova, A. M., Tserkovnogo, G. F. and Kaufman, B. D. (1963). *Morbidity and mortality from malignant neoplasms in the U.S.S.R.* English edition edited by J. G. Dean; Pitman Medical Publishing Co., London.

Ministry of Labour (1965). *Annual report of H.M. Chief Inspector of Factories on industrial health,* 1964. H.M. Stationery Office, London.

Mustacchi, P. and Shimkin, M. (1958). Cancer of the bladder and infestation with Schistosoma haematobium. *J. nat. Cancer Inst.,* **20,** 825.

Nielsen, A. and Clemmesen, J. (1957). Twin studies in the Danish Cancer Registry, 1942–55. *Brit. J. Cancer,* **11,** 327.

Pike, M. C., Williams, E. H. and Wright, B. (1967). Burkitt's tumour in the West Nile district of Uganda. *Brit. med. J.,* in press.

Pott, P. (1775). *Chirurgical observations relative to the cataract, the polypus of the nose, the cancer of the scrotum, the different kinds of ruptures, and the mortification of toes and feet.* London.

Sanghvi, L. D., Rao, K. C. M. and Khanolkar, V. M. (1955). Smoking and chewing of tobacco in relation to cancer of the upper alimentary tract. *Brit. med. J.,* **1,** 1111.

Satterlee, H. S. (1960). The arsenic poisoning epidemic of 1900: its relation to lung cancer in 1960, an exercise in retrospective epidemiology. *New Eng. J. Med.,***263,** 676.

Schwartz, D., Lellouch, J., Flamant, R. and Denoix, P. F. (1962). Alcool et cancer: résultats d'une enquête rétrospective. *Franc. Et. clin. biol.,* **7,** 590.

Segi, M. (1960). *Cancer mortality for selected sites in 24 countries* (1950–57). Department of Public Health, Tohoku University School of Medicine, Sendai, Japan.

Segi, M. and Kurihara, M. (1964). *Cancer mortality for selected sites in 24 countries, No. 3* (1960–1961). Department of Public Health, Tohoku University School of Medicine, Sendai, Japan.

Segi, M. and Kurihara, M. (1966). *Cancer mortality for selected sites in 24 countries, No. 4* (1962–1963). Department of Public Health, Tohoku University School of Medicine, Sendai, Japan.

Selikoff, I. J., Churg, J. and Hammond, E. C. (1964). Asbestos exposure and neoplasia. *J. Amer. med. Ass.*, **188,** 22.

Springett, V. H. (1966). The beginning of the end of the increase in mortality from carcinoma of the lung. *Thorax,* **21,** 132.

Steinitz, R. (1967). Uterine cancer. *Lancet,* **1,** 447.

Stewart, A. and Hewitt, D. (1963). Oxford survey of childhood cancers: progress report 1. *Monthly Bull. Minist. Hlth.*, **22,** 182.

Stewart, A., Webb, J. and Hewitt, D. (1958) A survey of childhood malignancies. *Brit. med. J.*, **1,** 1495.

Stocks, P. and Davies, R. I. (1964). Zinc and copper content of soils associated with the incidence of cancer of the stomach and other organs. *Brit. J. Cancer,* **18,** 14.

Tokuhata, G. K. and Lilienfeld, A. M. (1963). Familial aggregation of lung cancer in humans. *J. nat. Cancer Inst.*, **30,** 289.

United Nations Scientific Committee on the Effects of Atomic Radiation (1964). *General Assembly Official Records, Nineteenth Session.* United Nations, New York.

Verschuer, O. and Kober, E. (1956). Die Frage der erbli-
chen Disposition zum Krebs. Akademie der Wissen-
schaften und der hitteratur in Mainz; Steiner,
Wiesbaden.

Volkmann, R. (1874). On tar, paraffin, and soot cancer
(chimney sweepers' cancer). *Berlin klin. Wchnschr.*, **2,**
218.

Wagner, J. C. (1965). Epidemiology of diffuse mesothelial
tumours: evidence of an association from studies in
South Africa and the United Kingdom. *Ann. N.Y.
Acad. Sci.*, **132,** *575.*

Wallace, D. M. (1967). Bladder tumours in rubber workers
(discussion). *Proc. roy. Soc. Med.*, **60,** 16.

Wilson, S. R. (1910). *Report on mule-spinners' cancer.*
Manchester University, unpublished.

World Health Organization (1966). *World Health Statistics
Annual,* 1963. Vol. 1. Vital statistics and causes of
death. World Health Organization, Geneva.

Wright, D. H. (1966). Burkitt's tumour in England: a
comparison with childhood lymphosarcoma. *Int. J.
Cancer,* **1,** *503.*

Wynder, E. L. and Bross, I. J. (1961). A study of etiological
factors in cancer of the esophagus. *Cancer,* **14,** 389.

Wynder, E. L., Bross, I. J. and Day, E. (1956). A study of
environmental factors in cancer of the larynx. *Cancer,*
9, 86.

Wynder, E. L., Bross, I. J. and Feldman, R. M. (1957).
A study of etiological factors in cancer of the mouth.
Cancer, **10,** 1300.

Wynder, E. L. and Fairchild, E. P. (1967). Epidemiology
of persistent cough. *To be published.*

Yerushalmy, J. (1962). Statistical considerations and evaluation of epidemiological evidence. In: *Tobacco and Health*. Edited by G. James and T. Rosenthal; C. C. Thomas, Springfield, Illinois.

Yerushalmy, J. and Palmer, C. E. (1959). On the methodology of investigations of etiologic factors in chronic disease. *J. chron. Dis.*, **10, 27.**